The Whartons' Cardio-Fitness Book

Also by Jim and Phil Wharton

The Whartons' Stretch Book
The Whartons' Strength Book

The **Whartons'** Cardio-Fitness Book

The Step-by-Step Program for High Energy and Endurance

Jim and Phil Wharton

Authors of *The Whartons' Stretch Book*
and *The Whartons' Strength Book*

with Bev Browning

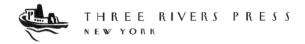
THREE RIVERS PRESS
NEW YORK

From out of pain to staying in the game, we salute you for enduring.
Keep pushing the high pace with us and loving it.
This book is for YOU.

Copyright © 2000 by Jim Wharton, Phil Wharton, and Maximum
Performance International, Inc.

All rights reserved. No part of this book may be reproduced or transmitted in any form or by any means, electronic or mechanical, including photocopying, recording, or by any information storage and retrieval system, without permission in writing from the publisher.

Published by Three Rivers Press, New York, New York. Member of the Crown Publishing Group.

Random House, Inc. New York, Toronto, London, Sydney, Auckland
www.randomhouse.com

THREE RIVERS PRESS is a registered trademark and the Three Rivers Press colophon is a trademark of Random House, Inc.

Printed in the United States of America

Design by Maggie Hinders

Library of Congress Cataloging-in-Publication Data

Wharton, Jim, 1940–
   The Whartons' cardio-fitness book : the step-by-step program for high energy and endurance / Jim and Phil Wharton.
   1. Heart—Diseases—Prevention.   2. Heart—Diseases—Exercise therapy.   3. Physical fitness.   I. Wharton, Phil, 1967–   II. Title.
   RC684.E9 W48 2000
   616.1'205—dc21   00-037725

ISBN 0-8129-3161-0

10 9 8 7 6 5 4 3 2 1

First Edition

Acknowledgments

Thank you so much to Michael Browning, who took us into his family while we worked with Bev to write this book. Many thanks to Reid Boates, the world's greatest agent, and Elizabeth Rapoport, the world's greatest editor. Thanks so much to Jim and Nancy Land of PDC, who build our books into joyful pages. Thank you to Allison Wagner, swimmer and U.S. Olympic silver medalist who designed the training program for swimming. Thank you to Jim Karanas, coholder of the world record in the 100-kilometer two-man tandem indoor rowing, for designing the training program for rowing. Thank you so much to Dr. Gabriele Rosa, athletic global director of the Fila Group and the medical director of the Marathon Clinic in Brescia, Italy, for his valuable insights into endurance training and rehabilitation. Thank you to the Kenyan runners who run for Fila, and train in Italy and Kenya. Special thanks to Moses Tanui and his wonderful family for welcoming Phil into their lives in Eldoret, Kenya, for two and a half months. Thank you, Philip Tanui, for Swami the Sheep. Many thanks to Loretta Rosa for her boundless enthusiasm and gracious hospitality, and for sharing her experience in running. Thank you to Claudio, Armando, Roberta, and Marco and Frederico Rosa in Italy. Thank you to running coaches and friends, Matt Centrowitz, Tom Craig, and Damian Koch. Thank you to the Lung Association of Arizona / New Mexico and the American Cancer Society for their valuable assistance in helping us research the effects of smoking and methods for quitting. Thank you to the Metropolitan Life Insurance Company for allowing us to reproduce their famous height and weight tables. Thank you for the generous personal contributions and support of Malcolm Privette, Dr. Dan Hamner, Jimmy Lynch, Mike Frankfurt, Hugh Hubbard, Shannon Silcox, Tom Nohilly, Salisha Abraham, and Michelle Assaf. Many thanks to Dr. Frank Rohter for his influence on endurance training and for teaching us all to live as athletes—"Outstanding!" Carol Gordon, without you, we would never leave the ground. You're the best.

And finally, we wish to thank our gentle friend Ron Boyle for his years of support and brotherhood. You will be missed.

Contents

Introduction

Jim and Phil Wharton, father and son, spend their professional lives working in their sports clinic in New York City. Because the sports clinic is tucked away on the ground floor of an unassuming building that overlooks the Museum of Natural History, no one would suspect that it's a center for training and rehabilitation for some of the most famous sports luminaries of our time. Men and women athletes from all over the world come to the Whartons when careers are on the line and performance is critical. The Whartons are familiar faces at Olympic competitions, world-championship track and swim meets, international aerobics competitions, baseball training camps, professional basketball- and football-team locker rooms, and backstage on Broadway. Their knowledge of the athlete's body is finely honed from years of experience and study. But more than that, their knowledge is personal. Both Whartons are accomplished distance runners. Clearly, when Jim or Phil takes an athlete's career in his hands, it's a case of "it takes one to know one." And no one knows the heart and soul of an athlete like a Wharton.

For several years, Jim and Phil have been working in Italy with Dr. Gabriele Rosa, the athletic global director for Fila. Dr. Rosa and his staff train marathon runners, among them the Kenyans who have dominated distance running for a long time. The Kenyan runners train in both the mountains of northern Italy and the high plains camps of Kenya. Phil, training under Dr. Rosa's watchful eye, had the opportunity to visit Kenya and train with some of the best runners in the world. Of course, Phil regarded this as an opportunity not only to advance his performance but to uncover the secrets that would unlock the mystery of the Kenyans. What are they doing that makes them best in the world? What magic do they possess that none of the rest of us have figured out yet? Over the course of a few months, Phil watched and listened. And finally figured it out.

Kenyans train by following the rhythms and cycles of nature. They rise in the morning and run as far and as fast as they can. Then they eat and rest for a long time, often going back to sleep. After they're rested, the cycle begins again. Like the lions and lionesses that share their high plains camps, the

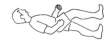

Kenyan runners pattern their lives in a fine balance between effort and rest. Of course. Why didn't we think of it sooner?

Phil and Jim Wharton have combined this simple principle with science to devise an endurance training pattern called "The Spiral Within a Spiral." It's not only natural, it's mathematical. Training that perfectly balances effort and rest is simply a matter of hard and easy workouts, within hard and easy days, within hard and easy weeks. As soon as you decide that it's time to get fit with the sound advice and coaching of the Whartons, your life will soon take an *upward* spiral.

How to Use This Book

We like to tell the story of the man who was walking along a riverbank when he noticed a drowning person tumbling along in the current. The man leaped into the river, pulled the drowning person to the bank, and continued his journey. A few minutes later, he saw another drowning person sweep by. Again he dove into the river, towed the drowning person to the bank, and continued his journey. Within a minute, yet another person swept by. This time, after the man had saved the third victim, he said to himself, "I can't keep leaping into the water to save these people. I need to walk upstream and stop whoever's throwing them into the river."

This story illustrates how we feel about heart disease. It's not enough to keep throwing medical resources at diseases that are caused by being inactive. We need to attack the problem at its source, which is no farther away than your couch. Simply put, we have become a nation of sitters. Nature didn't intend us to be sedentary, so when our bodies are inactive, life-threatening problems can set in. Here's how you can turn the situation around: get off your duff!

We've designed this book to be a reference for cardiovascular fitness with lots of information about your heart and how it functions, and what goes wrong and why—and more important, what you can do to get fit and healthy. The word "endurance" may conjure for you the image of someone climbing Everest—a journey fraught with pain and difficulty. When we talk about endurance, we're talking about the activities that keep us moving hard enough and long enough to strengthen our heart—and there's nothing painful or difficult about it. In fact, it's going to be fun.

To help you visualize the activities, we've included flip art along the sides of the pages that show the proper technique. You'll find relevant page numbers provided at the beginning of each activity section in Chapter 10.

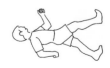

Cardio-Fitness Training Defined

When we think of cardio-fitness training, we usually think of this training as "aerobic"—meaning "living on air." Aerobic training, simply put, means that the activity demands oxygen. You breathe. So the point is to engage in an activity that gets your heart pumping and causes you to breathe more heavily, circulating oxygen and nutrients through your blood to all your cells, and strengthening your entire cardiovascular system. Although there are varying opinions on how often, how long, how much, and how hard, studies indicate that you need to work out with some degree of effort at least three to four times a week for at least thirty to forty-five minutes.

Although getting started is sometimes difficult, once you've had a small taste of feeling great, you won't have any trouble at all staying on your program. In fact, you're going to be so happy with the results that you'll soon be looking forward to your workouts with relish. You'll soon be trim, lean, energetic, and filled with the confidence that comes from control and accomplishment. But the outward changes tell only half the tale. The other even more important improvement will be to your cardiovascular system. The *Whartons' Cardio-Fitness Book* is a catalog of endurance activities carefully selected just for you:

Walking
Racewalking
Running
Jumping rope
Dancing
Swimming
In-line skating
Cross-country skiing
Cycling
Rowing

All you have to do is find the activity you like best, then follow the day-by-day training schedule we've designed to help you go from being sedentary to being lean, fit, energetic, and athletic in short order. Although we've outlined a training schedule that covers a full year, you'll feel better immediately. We'll keep you motivated and on track with tips and excuse busters you won't be able to refuse.

Like all the Whartons' athletes, you're about to embark on an adventure of self-discovery that will lead you to health and fitness. Let's get started!

Important Note: We are not physicians, and none of the advice in this book is intended to replace your doctor's advice; no book can do that. Before beginning this or any other fitness program, we strongly recommend that you share this book with your doctor so you can work together to improve your overall health.

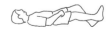

The Seven Myths About Endurance Training and Your Heart (the Myths You Must Never Repeat or Admit You Believed)

For as long as there have been athletes, the field of fitness has been rife with misconception, superstition, and myth. The confusion is understandable. The quest for excellence has always driven men and women to accept ideas—no matter how bizarre—that might give them "the edge," and to reject anything else—no matter how logical—that might threaten performance levels. Until a few years ago, when fitness found its way into the performance lab, the athlete's life was one of personal experimentation with heavy reliance on what other athletes or coaches suggested: the good, the bad, and the ugly. There's no question that "instinctive" approaches to training with shared information resulted in huge strides in performance in every sport. But we know now that most athletes who have gone before fell short of their potential, and a lot of people got hurt unnecessarily. Today, scientific and technological breakthroughs are providing new information to help us refine training and extend potential beyond anything our predecessors thought possible. Equally important, we now know that many of the ideas we had about human performance simply aren't true. We're debunking myths as fast as word will travel, but old beliefs are stubborn—especially those surrounding athletic performance and the human heart. Why? Because the consequence of being wrong can be a matter of life and death. If you make a mistake and put too much load on a knee, the consequence might be a strained knee. If you put too much load on a heart, the consequence might be a massive heart attack. In issues of mortality, the consensus is that it's better to be safe than sorry. Or is it? If being misinformed deprives you of a lifetime of fun and fitness, then you're not safe. You might even be at an increased risk of heart disease. Here are seven of the most common myths regarding exercise and the heart, and seven truths that challenge them.

MYTH 1.

If you've already had heart disease and exert yourself in any way, you'll have a heart attack, right?

WRONG!

Understandably, if you've been diagnosed with heart disease, or are recovering from a heart attack or open-heart surgery, you're likely to be concerned about putting stress on your heart. For many people, a heart problem is their first real face-to-face encounter with their own mortality. Disability or death is a frightening prospect that can cause you to conclude that you can't be too careful. But it might be foolish to avoid raising your heart rate ever again. Your heart problem didn't kill you. It was, in fact, your wake-up call to make some lifestyle changes and get into action. Rehabilitation should begin as soon as you are medically stabilized and feel well enough to begin, and your physician gives you the green light.

The world-famous Texas Heart Institute advises that the key to your rehabilitation and return to an active life "is improving your cardiovascular and physical conditioning . . . with a regular exercise routine that will develop the capacity of your heart and lungs, increase your flexibility, and gradually strengthen your muscles." Of course, your program—including everything in this book—must have your physician's full approval. When you begin exercise after a heart problem, it's only natural for you to be hypersensitive to every new sensation. After all, you're looking for symptoms that signal a recurrence of the problem. For example, when a healthy athlete feels out of breath, he probably will toss it off as just a little overexertion. In fact, he might even get excited at his effort and keep pushing, waiting for the second wind to kick in. You, on the other hand, might interpret being out of breath as a serious warning sign that you'll die if you take one more step. Experts in cardiology, while applauding vigilance, caution that emotional problems following the diagnosis of heart disease, or while recovering from a heart attack or open-heart surgery, can be as debilitating as the illness itself. If you're so afraid of dying that you stop living fully, then you need to alert your physician so he or she can help you find a counselor who specializes in dealing with your situation. A good rule of thumb is to regard your physician as your trusted partner in your health care. If the

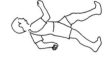

two of you have discussed your fitness program and your concerns, and you've been given the go-ahead, go ahead!

MYTH 2.

If your arteries are clogged and make your heart beat too fast, you'll have a stroke, right?

WRONG!

A stroke is a brain injury, or an "event," that happens when there's a hemorrhage in or around the brain, or when an artery is clogged with cholesterol, or when a small blood clot breaks loose from the wall of an artery and blocks blood flow to the brain. When blood can't get to the brain, the brain tissue is deprived of oxygen and the vital nutrients that blood carries, cells die, and physical and mental function are impaired. Because most of the culprits are blood clots and sticky cholesterol, it makes good sense that you should do everything possible to minimize your chances of developing either. Unless your physician advises you otherwise, exercise is critical. When the heart is not vigorously pumping, sluggish blood flow can increase the risk of a clot forming along the inner surface of the heart muscle itself. That's why people with impaired heart function are given anticoagulants to thin their blood. When you exercise regularly, your heart is stronger and more able to move blood so it's less likely to form clots. Your risk of stroke is decreased.

The role of healthy blood flow in controlling cholesterol is a little different. Here it's not a matter of keeping blood moving so much as it is a matter of using exercise to balance LDL (bad) and HDL (good) cholesterol. Increased levels of HDL are associated with decreased risk of cardiovascular disease. When LDL collects on artery walls and threatens to block blood flow, HDL comes along and lifts off particles of LDL and returns them to the liver. A low-fat, low-cholesterol diet and regular aerobic exercise can increase HDL levels and lower triglycerides.

Of course, if you have high cholesterol levels, or if you've ever experienced a blood clot, you need to check with your physician before you begin an exercise program.

MYTH 3.

An older person who starts exercising for the first time has to be extremely careful about shocking his or her system into a heart attack, right?

WRONG!

No matter how old you are, you should always get your physician's approval before you begin an exercise program. Of course, the older you are, the more cautious you are. And rightfully so. Not only have you had a longer time to develop a sedentary lifestyle, but you might have obvious, or not so obvious, health issues associated with aging that can impose limitations on your ability to work out.

We have one word of advice about shocking your system: don't. We insist that everyone exercise at his or her own pace. It's a simple judgment—when you feel comfortable, go for it. When you feel uncomfortable, back off or stop immediately. When we train a new runner and hear grumbling that one more lap around the track will surely result in a case of spontaneous human combustion, we reassure our client that nature imposes strict limits on the body in motion. You can do only what you can do. When your muscles, bones, connective tissue, and cardiovascular system can't support a hard workout, they all conspire to mandate an easy one. You slow down, whether or not you want to. No one we've trained has ever burst into flames (although Phil has come close).

We lose muscle mass at about 1 percent per year after age thirty. Additionally, we lose flexibility not only in connective tissues like tendons, but also in artery walls. This is called arteriosclerosis, or hardening of the arteries. Arteriosclerosis can cause blood pressure to rise and increase the heart's workload, causing the heart muscle itself to thicken and become less flexible. If you start an exercise program with those problems, you'll want to do so under a physician's supervision. But we also want to point out that these problems are among the strict limitations that nature imposes on your performance, like it or not. You don't have to worry about working out too hard, because frankly, it'll be impossible for you to exert that kind of effort. The point is that you work out at your own pace; you have no choice. And the more you work out, the longer you'll be able to work out the next time.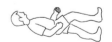

We assure you that the benefits will be well worth the time and energy you put into your program. Research conclusively demonstrates that people well into their nineties can make significant progress in regaining fitness levels in a relatively short period of time.

MYTH 4.

Being fat makes exercise dangerous. You should lose weight through dieting before you begin a fitness program, right?

WRONG!

With hundreds of diet books on the market and a wide selection of magazines featuring articles on weight loss every week, we are highly educated in the art and science of eating. Grocery-store shelves are lined with low-calorie, low-fat, and fat-free foods. The USFDA launched a nationwide educational initiative a few years ago to teach us all to read food labels, just like the scientists, so we can now ferret out the sugar and fat and make healthy choices in the grocery store. Anytime we turn on a television we can bet there'll be a program or an infomercial on weight loss. Among the most popular sites on the Internet are weight-loss programs, chat rooms, and support groups. Sales of pharmaceuticals that promise weight loss are at an all-time high. Diet programs like Jenny Craig and Weight Watchers are a multibillion-dollar industry. Hey, people, we *know* how to lose weight.

Or do we?

If we're such weight-loss experts, why are more than one third of all Americans obese? And how is it possible that that statistic is increasing yearly and exponentially, even among children?

We are fatter than ever because we have become a nation of sedentary people. It's as simple as that. Here's an easy physics lesson to help you understand what's happening here. The human body is thermodynamic, a sort of furnace that burns fuel (food) and converts it to energy. The amount of energy that each food has to release through this conversion is measured in *calories.* The rate at which the body uses the energy released by calories is measured by *metabolism.* Low metabolism means that the body can use only a little of the energy. High metabolism means that the body uses a lot. So let's put some simple principles together. If you eat more than you can use, you store the excess as fat, and gain weight. If you use more calories than you consume, your body uses what your last meal made available, then draws what it needs from storage. As your fat storage is depleted, you lose weight. If you really like consuming calories and are determined to eat more than you need at the moment, you can increase your ability to use them by revving up your metabolism with physical activity. Bottom line: we're getting fatter because we're storing energy that we're not using because we live in a society where many tasks are easier than nature intended them to be, and because we spend our free time sitting in front of televisions and computers.

To be fair and honest, we admit that you can lose weight temporarily by dieting alone. You can reduce your calories and force your body to draw from its fat storage, but unless you rev up your energy expenditure, you're doomed to gain weight again in pretty short order—as soon as you make the mistake of consuming more calories than you can use.

Unless you have a medical problem or are taking medication that causes weight gain, the answer is to get off your duff and use the energy your body has converted from the calories you've consumed. Here's a thought: try cutting back on your calories *and* revving up your energy expenditure. This way you'll create a double-whammy deficit, and one that will yield a quicker and more permanent weight loss. (By the way, if you've tried everything and still can't seem to get your weight under control, check with your physician. There are a number of medical and metabolic issues that might be hindering your best effort.)

The concern in starting an exercise program with a heavy person, of course, is that he or she suffers from structural problems caused by carrying so much weight. These concerns are well founded. We recommend that a heavy person (doctors define obesity as being 20 percent heavier than the ideal weight for your height) refrain from engaging in activity that unduly strains bones and connective tissues that are already under duress from excess weight. For example, we might suggest that a heavy person walk rather than run. Running will come later, after the weight drops off. Additionally, obesity can be accompanied by a number of other medical difficulties, such as diabetes. For this reason, it is imperative that if you are heavy, you get your physician's approval for any fitness activity.

MYTH 5.

Bypass surgery repairs a damaged heart and eliminates the need to exercise for cardiovascular fitness, right?

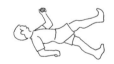

WRONG!

Bypass surgery doesn't cure coronary artery disease. It simply creates a detour for blood flow to the heart, bypassing blocked and damaged arteries. Bypassing does not eliminate the underlying cause of the blockages, like excess cholesterol that sticks to the artery walls and forms an ever-thickening plaque. In fact, the new grafted vessels can also succumb to disease within a few years if the heart patient can't get the disease under control with diet, exercise, and medications; patients sometimes have to repeat the bypass surgery. But surgeries cannot go on indefinitely, because surgeons will run out of blood vessels to harvest for the bypasses. If you've had a bypass and you're smart, you'll view the surgery as a second chance at life and make some serious changes in your lifestyle. The good news is that after a bypass, you'll likely feel stronger and more vigorous than you have in a long time. With renewed energy and commitment, you'll do well in the fitness program your physician approves.

MYTH 6.

Endurance exercise causes a lot of deaths. What about the famous runner and author Jim Fixx, who died on a run? Obviously, exerting yourself is risky, no matter how fit you are, right?

WRONG!

Exertion is risky when it triggers problems from an existing heart condition. Jim Fixx has been called the "Father of Running" in the United States, and is inarguably responsible for the 1970s running boom. His book put thousands of people into running shoes and propelled them out the front door. But Jim Fixx made a fatal mistake. He might have assumed that being physically fit assured perfect health. While we'll never really know what he was thinking, we do know that he ignored uncomfortable symptoms of heart disease and brushed off friends who advised him to get a stress test. He died on a run. A sport that had been touted as the perfect exercise for cardiovascular health had claimed a high-profile victim. Jim's death was a grim reminder that there are genetic and medical factors that running or any other endurance exercise can mitigate, but not overcome.

Heart problems and exertion are a potentially lethal combination. Physicians warn that risk is increased significantly when an untrained, unconditioned person suddenly takes on too much, too soon. Sound like a familiar scenario? It should. This is a classic example of the "weekend warrior"—a person who sits behind a desk all week, then rushes out on Saturday morning to play soccer or shovel snow. Statistically, fewer than 4 percent of all heart attacks appear to be triggered by exertion, but statistics don't matter at all if you're in that 4 percent. The moral of the story is that you should have yourself tested for preexisting medical problems before you begin an exercise program, get your physician's blessing, and train slowly. Advance in your activity only when your body can tolerate the effort. Go at your own pace, and you'll be fine.

MYTH 7.

Endurance exercise causes your heart to beat faster. Your heart will wear out sooner and you'll die younger if you exert yourself, right?

WRONG!

You'll die sooner if you don't exert yourself. Your heart is the most miraculous, dependable pump ever created. Without your having to think about it, by the end of a normal life span, it will have beaten 3.5 billion times . . . plenty of beats to keep you alive, no matter how active you are. Your heart muscle, unlike other muscles, doesn't tire out. It does become less efficient, beating too slowly or too quickly, only when it's injured, diseased, or disrupted electrically. In other words, unless something catastrophic happens, you can count on it. When you exert effort, nature has designed your heart to pump faster to carry blood with oxygen and nutrients to your cells, then flush away metabolic waste products generated during that effort. When the effort is over, your heart returns to its normal pace within a few minutes. It's all part of the grand design. Exercise—getting your heart rate up—doesn't wear your heart out. On the contrary, regular exercise makes your heart stronger, more efficient, and healthier. Regular exercise also conditions your whole body. Strong muscles, particularly the large muscles like your quadriceps, actually assist the heart in maintaining efficient blood flow.

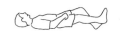

PART ONE

The Healthy Heart

1.

An Owner's Quick Guide to the Cardiovascular System

For as long as there have been human beings, there has been a collective understanding that the human heart is somehow at the center of all life in a spiritual, emotional, and mystical sense. When we love someone, we express it as "I love you with all my heart." When we are despondent, we are "brokenhearted." When we fully grasp a situation, we say, "I know it in my heart." When we've been terribly disappointed, we say, "It tore my heart out." When we speak of the absolute core of an issue, it's called "the heart of the matter." When we are affirming intuition, we say, "What does your heart tell you to do?" or "Did you follow your heart?" We could go on and on with "heartisms," but the point is that the heart is unquestionably more than an organ that pumps blood. The human spirit recognizes it as life force. If you doubt our observation, try transposing any other vital organ with "heart" in one of these expressions and you'll understand (after you stop laughing). "I love you with all my spleen" and "I am broken livered" just don't make the point, do they?

We recognize the importance of "heart" in the world of professional and amateur sports. When we speak of an athlete in terms of heart, we refer to the courage, discipline, and tenacity of that individual. But we also acknowledge that the heart—the physical heart—is critical to the foundation of training. More important, it's critical to good health and well-being. For this reason, all training begins with cardiovascular fitness. The ability to oxygenate the body, carry and deliver nutrients, and flush waste products is the responsibility of the heart. And it does a miraculous job.

One beat at a time, your heart beats 100,000 times per day, and pumps about 2,000 gallons of blood. You don't have to think about it. It's set on autopilot, adjusting its own pace to meet the demands you place on it. Running through the yard after your dog? Need more oxygen? Your heart will speed up. Sprawled out, snoozing on the floor in the den? Need less oxygen? Your heart will slow down. Over your lifetime, it will pump more than 50 million gallons of blood as you work hard and rest easy . . . and everything in between.

CARDIOLOGY 101—WHARTON STYLE

The anatomy, physiology, and function of the heart are complex, but we're going to attempt to explain it all in a few short sentences. Basically, the heart is a pump about the size of your fist, located in the middle of your upper chest, just left of your sternum (breastbone). It is made up of four chambers, two on each side. Each of the upper chambers is called an atrium. Each of the lower chambers is called a ventricle. The upper chambers—the atria—receive blood from veins. You might have noticed that some of the blood vessels you can see through your skin appear to be blue. You're observing veins carrying blood devoid of oxygen and being returned to the heart. That venous blood has taken a side trip through your liver, an elegant filter that removes metabolic by-products and toxins. Once the blood gets back to the heart, the ventricles take over. The right ventricle pumps blood through pulmonary arteries to the lungs, where it will be oxygenated and returned to the heart. (When the blood picks up oxygen, it turns bright red again.) The left ventricle sends that oxygenated blood through arteries out to the body, including down through your spleen, which filters out damaged blood cells, and your kidneys, which filter toxins to be eliminated in urine. Strong valves keep the blood moving in the right direction, in the right sequence, and under the proper pressure. The sound you hear when you listen to a heart—*lub-dub, lub-dub*—is made by the valves as they open and close. While the heart is receiving blood and sending it

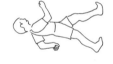

back out to the lungs and the rest of the body, it receives its own special blood supply from the aorta, through coronary arteries.

As an athlete, you need to be aware that your heart is at the center of your life force and physical power. It's a muscle that, like all others, you must condition. Your ability to perform is directly related to its strength and health. Building the heart muscle to support your workouts will take time. Fortunately, cardiac conditioning will take place as you train your body to adapt to your activity. And the benefits of a healthy, strong heart are legion. Having a healthy heart will add quality to your life and quantity to your years.

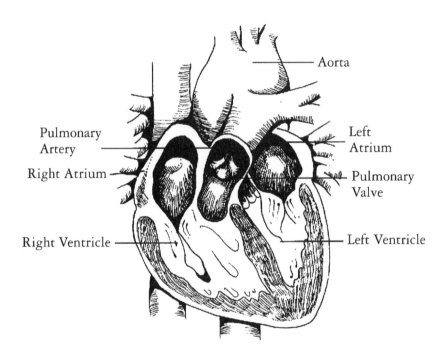

2.
Diseases You Might Be Able to Head Off If You're Heart-Smart

The U.S. Surgeon General has listed a sedentary lifestyle as one of the top killers in our country. If sloth is a killer, the killer has five henchmen that form the World's Most Unwanted List: coronary artery disease, diabetes, high cholesterol, hypertension, and stroke. This lineup of deadly conditions that are directly related to inactivity should be enough to scare anyone off the couch! Fortunately, you can largely prevent or minimize the damage with even a moderate program of regular physical exercise. You don't have to be an Olympian or quit your job to devote yourself to the gym. All you have to do is eat a healthy diet and get off your duff a few times a week for thirty minutes at a time. It couldn't be easier or more fun. Let's review the killers for a little motivation:

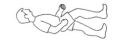

KILLER NUMBER 1—CORONARY ARTERY DISEASE

When we hear about coronary artery disease, this refers to blockages in this specific system of arteries. The blockages can be caused by plaque or blood clots—we'll give you plenty of detail on that later in this chapter. When arteries are blocked and unable to supply blood to the heart muscle, the heart is damaged or dies, and a heart attack is triggered.

An Aspirin a Day to Protect Your Heart

Run-of-the-mill aspirin may be one of the most potent heart protectors we have, since it helps to thin the blood and prevents clogging of the blood vessels. Researchers tell us that taking between one and six aspirins a week lowers the risk of having a heart attack, and confers a decrease in risk for a second heart attack or stroke.

Now that doesn't mean you should start taking aspirin on your own; after all, this common pain reliever can actually cause some serious side effects, such as ulcers and stomach bleeding. If you'd like to try it, consult your physician first to make sure aspirin therapy is safe and smart for you, and to determine how much you should take. (Those who shouldn't take aspirin include people with blood-clotting disorders, ulcers, and asthma.)

KILLER NUMBER 2—DIABETES

Diabetes is a metabolic disorder that disrupts your body's ability to convert food into energy. When you eat food, your body converts most of it through digestion into glucose, a simple sugar transported through the bloodstream to cells that use it for energy, growth, and repair. The transfer of perfect amounts of glucose from the blood to your cells is regulated and facilitated by insulin, a miraculous hormone produced in your pancreas. Diabetes is characterized by disruption and disturbance of your body's ability to produce or use insulin. Without insulin, or with insufficient amounts of insulin, your body is unable to transfer glucose to the cells, so the glucose stays in your bloodstream, eventually building up until it overflows into the urine and is excreted. As a consequence, your cells never receive the energy they need to sustain life as you know it.

The Centers for Disease Control reports that 15.7 million people, or 5.9 percent of the U.S. population, suffer from diabetes, but only two thirds of these know it. There are several types of diabetes:

Type 1 diabetes—called insulin-dependent diabetes mellitus, or juvenile-onset diabetes. Risk factors are not as well defined as with other types of diabetes, but autoimmune, genetic, and environmental factors contribute.

Type 2 diabetes—also called non-insulin-dependent diabetes mellitus, or adult-onset diabetes. Risk factors include aging, obesity, family history of diabetes, prior history of gestational diabetes, impaired glucose tolerance, physical inactivity, and race/ethnicity. At particular risk are Native Americans and Americans of African, Hispanic/Latino, and Asian origin.

Gestational diabetes—this disease develops in a small percentage of pregnant women, but usually disappears spontaneously when the pregnancy is over. Gestational diabetes occurs most frequently in Native Americans, and Americans of African and Hispanic/Latino origin. Women who experience it are at increased risk of developing Type 2 diabetes later in their lives.

Other specific types—a small percentage develops from genetic syndromes, surgery, medications, malnutrition, infections, and other illnesses.

Complications from diabetes can be debilitating. In fact, the disease can be fatal. Adults with diabetes are two to four times more likely to die of heart disease than adults without diabetes. Their risk of stroke is two to four times greater. Between 60 and 65 percent of all adults with diabetes have high blood pressure. Diabetes is the leading causes of blindness and end-stage kidney disease in adults. More than half of all people with diabetes have some form of damage to the nervous system, including numbness or pain in extremities, and impaired digestion in the stomach lining. More than half of the amputations of lower limbs in the United States occur in patients with diabetes. Also, periodontal disease occurs in 30 percent of all diabetic adults. Diabetes in pregnant women can cause birth defects and fetal death. And diabetes can induce life-threatening comas.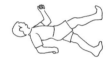

The treatments for diabetes are advancing rapidly through research. Managing Type 1 diabetes requires a daily balanced program of diet, exercise, glucose testing, and insulin injections. Managing Type 2 diabetes follows the same program, except that insulin injections might be unnecessary. Almost 90 percent of all people with Type 2 diabetes are overweight, and most are over age forty. In many cases, Type 2 can be controlled exclusively with diet and exercise: getting the weight off and getting the disease under control. Of course, it's logical that Type 2 diabetes can be largely prevented by maintaining a normal weight: a combination of eating a healthy diet and getting regular exercise.

Exercise is a vital part of preventing and managing diabetes. Regular, vigorous physical activity assists insulin's effectiveness so cells can more easily absorb glucose, lowers glucose levels in the blood, and increases the strength of your heart to help circulate blood through the smaller vessels and keep extremities from suffering diminished blood supply. Additionally, exercise will help keep your weight under control.

If you are on insulin, the timing of your workout in relationship to your meals will be important. Your physician can help you refine scheduling to balance eating with working out. If you're working out more than an hour after a meal, you might first eat a snack that will fuel the type of workout you're planning. Moderate workout: lead off with a light, high-carbohydrate snack. Heavier, more advanced workout: add a little protein to the high-carbohydrate snack, and eat a more generous portion. If the workout is going to be a long one, or if your blood-sugar level is low, you might need to take a break and eat a snack mid-workout. If you experience an insulin reaction while working out—feeling faint, dizzy, or confused, or sweating more than you think is normal—stop the workout immediately and get some glucose into your system. Also, it's a good idea to let your workout partner know that you have diabetes and how he or she can help you if your blood-sugar level drops too low.

If you have diabetes, it is imperative that you consult your physician before designing your workout program and organizing your diet.

KILLER NUMBER 3—HIGH CHOLESTEROL

In spite of the media war against it, cholesterol doesn't fully deserve the bad rap it's taken. We're all frantically trying to get the numbers as low as possible and cut it out of our diets entirely. But if you never ate another molecule of cholesterol, your body would happily continue to produce it for you and release it into your bloodstream. Your body needs it. Cholesterol is a necessary component in our cell walls. Our glands use it to manufacture hormones. And it assists the liver in making bile, used to digest fats.

The Good, the Bad, and the Ugly

So why is cholesterol considered such a killer if it's so necessary? Cholesterol is an oily, waxy, fatty substance that circulates through the body in blood. Blood is water-based, and everyone knows oil and water don't mix. To protect the cholesterol molecule from damage, the body coats it with a sort of waterproof protein that allows it to navigate through the bloodstream without getting wet. This little package shooting the rapids is called a lipoprotein.

Most cholesterol is LDL, or low-density lipoprotein, nicknamed "bad" cholesterol. It's closely associated with risk of cardiovascular disease. In high concentrations, it tends to stick to the artery walls and slowly build up over time.

This sticky buildup is called plaque. Eventually, when the plaque is thick enough, it will clog off the artery, shutting down blood flow.

But not all cholesterol is considered bad. HDL, high-density lipoprotein, is called the "good" cholesterol, a well-deserved reputation. Increased levels of HDL are associated with decreased risk of cardiovascular disease. Why? Because as LDL is collecting on artery walls and threatening to block blood flow, HDL comes along and lifts off particles of LDL and returns them to the liver. It's a classic case of good versus evil, where virtue triumphs and the patient lives.

Cholesterol: Check It Out with Checkups

Have your LDL, HDL, and total cholesterol levels checked regularly. These are numbers you need to know. The procedure is a simple blood test. We recommend that you have the tests done by your physician, and urge you not to rely on finger-prick tests that are popular at health fairs or in home kits.

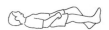

The magic number (established for both men and women by research consensus) for your total cholesterol is 200. Anything above 200 is considered to be a warning sign that you're at increased risk of developing cardiovascular disease. This doesn't mean that you *will* develop disease. You're just at risk. Conversely, having a number below 200 doesn't guarantee immunity from cardiovascular disease; you've just got a statistical advantage. The higher the number, the higher the risk. The lower the number, the lower the risk.

Remember that 200 is the composite of HDL and LDL levels. There are two more numbers within the number that you need to know. Physicians recommend that if your total cholesterol is below 200, you need not concern yourself with specifics of the composites. You can relax. But if your total cholesterol is above 200, you'll want to know levels of both HDL and LDL, because here's where the good and the bad can turn ugly.

In both men and women with a total cholesterol level of 200 or less, the LDL level should be less than 130, and the HDL level should be 60 or more. Don't worry about having to conduct an algebraic analysis of your lab report with a calculator. You can count on your physician to review the results of your cholesterol test with you and make recommendations.

If you're concerned about lowering your LDL levels, there are many things you can do to help.

1. *Eat a balanced diet low in fat and high in soluble and insoluble fiber.* You'll not only be able to lower your cholesterol levels by as much as 10 percent, but you might have the added bonus of weight loss.

2. *If you smoke, quit right this second.* Don't even finish reading this list before you get up and throw away your cigarettes. You've known all along that smoking causes lung cancer. Now we're telling you that it impedes the production of HDL, the cholesterol you need to combat cardiovascular disease. Additionally, smoking increases the risk of blood clots. In other words, smoking increases your risk of heart disease. The combination of clogged arteries and blood clots is a double whammy you simply do not want to deal with.

3. *If you drink alcohol, do so in moderation.* Interesting studies indicate that moderate alcohol consumption can help raise HDL. Some of these studies have centered specifically around red wines and decreased risk of cardiovascular disease. No matter what the benefit, a little bit of alcohol goes a long way. Increased consumption of alcohol has its own health risks, so practice moderation. If you don't drink now, don't start. It's not necessary. Check in with your doctor about drinking.

4. *Exercise.* Congratulations—you're reading the right book. Studies conclude that regular aerobic exercise increases HDL levels and lowers triglycerides (fats in your blood). Your added bonus will be a fit, trim body.

5. *You can take medications to lower cholesterol levels and control triglycerides.* Your physician will likely recommend this only after you have attempted to bring your levels into a healthy range through diet, exercise, smoking cessation, and alcohol moderation . . . and failed.

Remember that cholesterol is only one piece of a puzzle that comes with no guarantees. You can do everything right and still develop cardiovascular disease. And we've all met people who do everything wrong, yet enjoy long lives. But it's important not to assume that life is a game of chance, where you have no control. In fact, you do have a great deal of control. Use education and discipline to tip the statistics in your favor. Take charge of all aspects of your health, including controlling cholesterol.

KILLER NUMBER 4—HYPERTENSION (HIGH BLOOD PRESSURE)

Blood pressure is a general term that describes two forces working in concert: one is the force created by the heart as it pumps blood through the arteries, and the other is the force of the arteries as they resist. Blood pressure is expressed as two numbers, one over the other. The top number is "systolic": the pressure of the heart while compressing to beat or pump. The lower number is "diastolic": the pressure of the heart while resting between beats. When you hear a blood pressure reading, you'll always hear the systolic pressure given first, followed by the diastolic pressure. For example, a reading of 110/70 (pronounced "110 over 70") means that the systolic pressure is 110 and the diastolic pressure is 70. So how do we interpret blood pressure?

Lower than 140/90—good

Exactly 140/90—a little high; would need periodic checking

Greater than 140/90—high

As a general rule for a healthy person, the lower the blood pressure, the better—unless low pressure starts triggering symptoms like light-headedness. If your blood pressure does register as high, it doesn't necessarily mean you have high blood pressure, because there are a lot of factors and circumstances that can affect a single reading. But a reading that indicates high blood pressure should put you on alert. You'll want to get it checked again, and soon.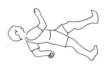

High blood pressure is called hypertension. Even though the word implies tension, it's not referring to a relationship between blood pressure and your state of mind. You can be calm, cool, and collected—and still have hypertension. On the flip side, you can be a nervous wreck and have low blood pressure. Usually (and if you're lucky) the first time you might discover that you have high blood pressure is in your physician's office with a cuff on your arm. Although one out of four adults has it, many people are unaware until they are told or until something catastrophic happens. Generally, hypertension has no symptoms. This is why it's called the silent killer. The American Heart Association reports that hypertension, no matter how silent, directly increases the risk of coronary heart disease (which leads to heart attack) and stroke.

Although hypertension can be the direct result of an existing medical condition like diabetes or kidney disease, in more than 90 percent of all cases, the causes are not specifically understood. The good news is that the condition is easy to detect and usually can be controlled. Researchers might not be clear about the causes, but they do know that certain types of people are at greater risk for developing hypertension: people whose parents had hypertension, males, people who are sensitive to the effects of salt, African-Americans, Hispanics, middle-aged and elderly people, obese people, sedentary people, people under prolonged stress, heavy drinkers, women on oral contraceptives, and patients with diabetes, gout, or kidney disease. Additionally, statistics suggest that the lower the educational and income levels of a person, the greater the risk of hypertension. By the way, if you think adults on this alarming list are the only people at risk for developing high blood pressure, think again. Kids can also fall victim. There are a lot of factors that are absolutely out of your control, but a quick scan of the list will reveal that there is a lot you *can* do to prevent hypertension. Incidentally, smoking isn't listed as a risk factor in developing hypertension, but it does decrease the effects of medications your physician might have to prescribe. And smoking does put you at risk of other medical horrors we all know well, such as cancer, gastric ulcers, chronic bronchitis, and emphysema.

So what's the big deal? Elevated blood pressure is an indication that the heart and arteries are working much harder than they should. Over time, the heart will enlarge to try to meet the increasing demands of its own inefficiency. Damage will set in. The arteries will become hardened, scarred, and less elastic. This is called atherosclerosis. At best, damaged arteries are increasingly unable to transport blood to supply the body's organs and tissues with nutrients and oxygen. In turn, systems start to fail. At worst, damaged arteries narrow until they completely block blood supply to vital organs: the heart, brain, and kidneys. The result can be heart attack, stroke, and kidney disease. In extreme circumstances, an artery might bulge (aneurysm) or burst (hemorrhage) from the overload. Combine hypertension with high cholesterol, and you have double trouble. There is conclusive evidence that when both blood pressure and cholesterol are elevated, the risk of cardiovascular disease is exponential.

Lowering blood pressure that's too high is sometimes a simple matter of getting active and losing a few pounds of fat. Studies link obesity (over 20 percent above ideal weight) with hypertension (or at least a gradual elevation in pressure to higher ranges of "normal" as pounds increase over time). No matter what you weigh, if you've been diagnosed with hypertension and are otherwise healthy, one of the first things your physician will do is put you on a program of regular exercise that gets your heart rate up. A medically prescribed fitness program's goals are to lower blood pressure, raise levels of HDL (good) cholesterol that carries away artery-clogging LDL, burn fat, develop muscle, and strengthen your cardiovascular system. A wonderful side effect, of course, is that you're going to look and feel great in short order.

Other ways that your physician might manage hypertension include helping you make dietary changes (like losing your salt shaker and bypassing processed foods), limiting dietary cholesterol and saturated fats, putting you on a smoking cessation program, and, as a last resort, prescribing medications. In addition, you'll want to have your blood pressure checked at intervals your physician suggests.

KILLER NUMBER 5—STROKE

A stroke is a brain injury or an "event" that happens when a small blood clot or a bit of cholesterol breaks loose from the wall of an artery and clogs blood flow. It can happen several ways and from several sites. For example, the blood clot or cholesterol debris might break loose in the carotid artery in the neck and enter the bloodstream, where it's swept along toward the brain. As the branches of the artery become smaller and smaller, the clot or cholesterol debris 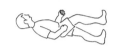 becomes wedged, blocking the blood flow to the brain. Brain cells die when they no longer receive oxygen and nutrients from blood. This is the stroke. But the clots or cholesterol debris don't have to break loose and travel to cause a stroke. They can stay where they are, increase in size until blood flow is squeezed off, and cause a stroke. A stroke also can be caused just by bleeding in and around the brain. Nothing suggests that the faster the blood flow, the greater the risk. To the contrary, having a strong, fit heart is one way to avoid problems.

Because the culprits are blood clots and sticky cholesterol, it makes good sense that you should do everything possible to minimize your chances of developing either. Exercise is critically important. When the heart is not vigorously pumping, sluggish blood flow can cause clots, increasing the risk that a clot will form along the inner surface of the heart muscle itself. That's why people with impaired heart function are given anticoagulants to thin their blood. When you exercise regularly, your heart is strong and vigorous and keeps blood flowing so it doesn't have a chance to form clots. Your risk of stroke is decreased.

The role of blood flow in controlling cholesterol is a little different. Here it's not a matter of keeping blood moving so much as it is a matter of using exercise to balance cholesterol. To sum it all up, you want your LDL (bad) cholesterol down and your HDL (good) cholesterol up. How? Among other things, lower the cholesterol and fat in your diet to help get LDL under control. And get off your duff. Regular aerobic exercise increases HDL levels and lowers triglycerides.

3.
Assessing Your Risk of Cardiovascular Disease

No discussion of cardiovascular fitness would be complete without mentioning the role that genetics plays in your biological makeup. If you thought that the extent of your family resemblance was limited to Mom's hair and Dad's nose, think again. Not only did you inherit unmistakable physical attributes from your parents (attractive, right?), but you also inherited nearly seventy thousand genes that are responsible for more than four thousand identifiable traits.

The link between genetics and heart disease is well documented. In fact, if one of your parents, grandparents, or siblings had early onset of heart disease (before age fifty-five), then your physician will automatically note that you have a major risk factor in developing heart disease yourself. (Another commonly inherited disease is high cholesterol—familial hypercholesterolemia, or FH. One out of every five hundred people in the world inherits the disease . . . and the other four hundred and ninety-nine aren't feeling all that secure either.) Don't blame your family and their irresponsible, hard-livin' ways for your newfound risk factor. It's not their fault. They, too, inherited the genetic encoding that predisposes them to heart disease. In spite of this shared problem, there is one way that you and your parents and grandparents are *not* alike. They probably didn't know they were at risk. You do. This knowledge gives you a measure of control that your parents never had. Geneticists tell us that some of the big killers—like heart disease—are the function of genetics working in cahoots with lifestyle factors, like diet. In other words, if you have a genetic predisposition for heart disease, it's a good bet that there are precautions you can take to help prevent it. Diet, exercise, health, and stress management might give you an edge.

YOUR ROOTS

For reasons that are not yet clearly understood, some forms of cardiovascular disease are statistically significant in some racial and ethnic groups in the

United States. While scientists attempt to sort genetics from geography, customs, and socioeconomic factors that might contribute, one thing is clear. There are differences. Compared to the total population, African-American men and women are at increased risk of coronary heart disease. On the other hand, Hispanic males have a 35 percent lower incidence of death from cardiovascular diseases, and Hispanic women have a 20 percent lower incidence.

BODY SHAPE: WHERE YOUR GENES FIT INTO YOUR JEANS

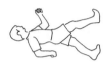

Look no farther than your fruit bowl to examine an important genetic attribute: your shape. For reasons of simplicity in describing the storage of excess body fat, the scientific community has divided us all into two categories: apples and pears (although anyone who knows Jim Wharton would insist on a third category—string bean). If you store body fat around your middle, as most men do, you're an "apple." If you store body fat in your hips, buttocks, and thighs, then you're a "pear." The significance of these designations, besides aesthetic, is that the apple-shaped people—both men and women—may be at higher risk of heart disease. Researchers are not yet clear about the reasons for this increased risk, but it's possible that excess fat around the waist influences cholesterol levels. And some physicians think that this concentration of fat in closer proximity to the heart might somehow place additional strain on it.

How do you know whether you're a pear or an apple? It's easy to tell. Merely remove your clothing and examine yourself in a full-length mirror. Turn to the side, then turn completely around to have a look at your backside from over your shoulder. That which disappears in the front view might be clearly visible from another point of view. A "gut" that hangs over a man's belt is an apple clue. Wide hips below a narrow waist is a pear clue. If you are still unclear (or can't believe your eyes), get out the tape measure. Measure your waist while you are standing—no cheating by sucking in your stomach or cinching the tape measure until you turn blue! Then measure your hips at the widest point of your buttocks. You can find this point by slipping the tape measure down, and letting it out gradually as you go. When the measure goes suddenly slack and even drops, you've just passed your widest circumference. Back up to it. Again, no cheating. Divide your waist measurement by your hip measurement to get your waist-to-hip ratio. An apple's ratio is greater than one. A pear's ratio is less than one.

So what's the significance of your body shape? Apples, beware! In a woman, a waist-to-hip ratio greater than 80 percent means that she is at increased risk of heart disease. In other words, she's carrying too much excess fat, and in the wrong place—her middle. In a man, a waist-to-hip ratio greater than 95 percent means that he, too, is at increased risk of heart disease. In other words, he's an apple guy carrying his excess fat in the middle. Not good.

You inherited your apple or pear shape, or at least your tendency to deposit fat in one of these two patterns that have been in your family for generations. But knowing what you now know, it's absolutely your responsibility to reshape your body to a more healthy ratio. Diet and exercise are the keys to success. If you've discovered a rotten apple in your basket, this is one genetic predisposition to cardiovascular disease you can control. Yes, indeed.

SETTING THE RECORD STRAIGHT

By the way, denial is not effective in dealing with genetic predisposition to cardiovascular disease. What you don't know *can* hurt you. You should be as informed as possible regarding your family's medical history, and you should pass that information on to your physician to insert into your permanent medical records. This is one case where bad news might really work to your advantage and even help save your life.

With regard to your significant cardiovascular genetic blueprint, here's what your physician will want to know about you.

HAS ANYONE IN YOUR FAMILY EVER HAD:

Coronary heart disease?	High cholesterol levels?
Congestive heart failure?	Vascular disease (such as
Cardiomyopathy?	atherosclerosis)?
Theumatic heart disease?	Diabetes?
Arrhythmias?	Hypertension?
Sudden death?	Stroke?

RISK FACTORS: LUCK OF THE DRAW OR STYLE OF YOUR LIFE?

Genetics notwithstanding, some people are more at risk for cardiovascular diseases than others. Researchers have developed a list of factors that increase the statistical probability that a person will develop the diseases. As you scan the list, be aware that you can have some of the risk factors and never have a problem. Or you can have none of the risk factors and still develop cardiovascular disease. Notice also that many of these risk factors are lifestyle-related and under your control. You can eliminate or lessen a risk factor by changing your behavior. As always, we insist that you discuss your concerns and plans with your physician.

Age. Statistically, the risk of cardiovascular disease increases as you grow older, perhaps because the connective tissues in artery walls become less flexible as we age. As the arteries' efficiency decreases, blood pressure tends to elevate and force the heart to work harder. Eventually, muscle tissue in the heart becomes damaged.

Gender. Cardiovascular disease is the leading cause of death in both men and women. Men are more likely to die of the disease at an earlier age than women, but as both genders get older, women catch up statistically. Menopause seems to be a turning point. As estrogen production ceases, women lose the cardio-protective properties of this hormone. In younger men and women, the only time both genders are at equal risk is when diabetes and high cholesterol are present.

Cholesterol and triglyceride levels. People with total cholesterol levels over 240 are at more than twice the risk of people with cholesterol levels below 200. If your cholesterol levels are below 200, before you relax and dive into a bag of chips, remember that this number is a composite of several measures. Knowing specific levels of LDL, HDL, and triglycerides (fats circulating in your blood) will still be important. Your physician will interpret the numbers for you and make recommendations. You can do plenty of things to control cholesterol and triglyceride levels: lower the saturated fat and cholesterol in your diet, get active, and, if you're a woman past menopause, consider hormone replacement therapy. If you can't lower your levels of cholesterol and triglyceride, your physician can prescribe medications to help.

Blood pressure. Even mildly elevated blood pressure and cardiovascular disease go hand in hand. The higher the pressure, the greater the risk of heart attack, atherosclerosis, and stroke. There is much you can do to lower your blood pressure with exercise and diet. For every five to six points you reduce your pressure, the risk of heart disease declines by 20 to 25 percent and the risk of stroke by 30 to 40 percent.

Cigarette smoking. If you smoke, your risk of dying of coronary artery disease is three times greater than your risk of dying of lung cancer. You're twice as likely to suffer a heart attack as a nonsmoker, and you're more likely to die within the hour. If you're a woman on oral contraceptives, you're nearly forty times more likely to have a heart attack than a nonsmoking woman. Quit immediately.

Physical activity. The U.S. Surgeon General has designated a sedentary lifestyle as hazardous to your health. It's a killer, equal in risk to hypertension, high cholesterol, and smoking. Getting off the couch and out the door into a program of regular physical activity is fully in your control.

Early menopause. Women who experience menopause before age forty-five—either surgically or spontaneously—have a slightly increased risk of developing cardiovascular diseases because they lose the cardioprotective benefits of estrogen earlier. The earlier the onset of menopause, the greater the risk.

Diabetes. Both insulin-dependent and non-insulin-dependent diabetes increase the risk of cardiovascular disease in men and women. Both genders are at particular risk of developing atherosclerosis at an earlier age than people who don't have diabetes, and the blockages tend to be more aggressive. More than 80 percent of people with diabetes die of some sort of cardiovascular disease.

Weight. Obesity—carrying too much body fat—increases risk of cardiovascular disease, even if no other risk factors are present. Obesity is defined as being more than 20 percent above normal weight for someone your age, gender, and height. Some studies suggest that even modest amounts of weight gained in the middle years double the risk. Carrying extra weight puts an increased load on the heart and increases blood pressure, triglyceride levels, and your risk of developing non-insulin-dependent diabetes. Eating a healthy diet and getting regular exercise to burn fat are in your control.

Stress. Scientists are not yet willing to conclude that stress and cardiovascular disease are linked, but they have strong suspicions. Stress triggers a physiological reaction in the endocrine system known as the fight or flight response, nature's miraculous way of getting you "battle-ready." Your adrenal glands go into overdrive to produce hormones that increase your heart rate, accelerate your breathing, raise your blood pressure, release fats into your blood, and rocket blood-sugar levels. The hormones even increase the stickiness of your platelets, so that your blood will clot more easily. Your body is prepared to take on the enemy or run like the wind. But what happens if the stress is merely emotional and your body never gets into action? And what happens if you throw your system into battle-ready constantly? Evidence suggests that constant stress might cause chronic increases in heart rate, blood pressure, and cholesterol levels. Also, scientists have found a strong correlation between certain personality traits and the incidence of heart diseases. People—men in particular—who are competitive, aggressive, hostile, impatient, and urgent about time are more likely to have heart attacks than their easygoing counterparts.

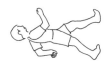

High levels of stored iron. Increased storage of iron in the body appears to increase risk of cardiovascular disease. In fact, in men, iron storage might be a risk factor more significant than high cholesterol, hypertension, or even diabetes. The release of excess iron appears to contribute to the formation of oxygen-free radicals that oxidize LDL cholesterol so that it sticks to artery walls and forms plaque more easily. Also the ferritin (stored iron) molecules release iron into tissue that has been injured, which could cause even more damage to the heart muscle following a heart attack. In a five-year study of men, scientists were able to associate that for every 1 percent increase in serum ferritin above normal levels, there was a 4 percent increase in risk of heart attack. More than 200 micrograms of serum ferritin per liter of blood doubled the risk. Stored iron could be one of the reasons that women experience an increase in risk of cardiovascular disease after menopause. When women cease to menstruate, they store excess levels of iron. But don't just throw away your iron supplements; speak to your physician first.

High levels of fibrinogen. Fibrinogen is a coagulant, meaning it helps blood clot so you won't bleed to death when you're cut. High levels of this coagulant—and the consequent increase in the tendency toward blood clots—have been associated with an increased risk of cardiovascular disease in men. Happily, levels of fibrinogen are reduced with regular physical exercise.

Male pattern baldness. This is a hereditary condition of hair loss triggered by high levels of the hormone androgen. Men lose hair from the front of the scalp over the crown of the head, forming a sort of horseshoe pattern of hair from one ear around the back of the head to the other ear. Some studies suggest that men with male pattern baldness also experience slightly increased risk of cardiovascular disease. (Even though women also inherit a form of pattern baldness, there is little evidence of any link between this and cardiovascular disease.)

Deficiency in B vitamins. Studies have linked risk of cardiovascular disease with deficiencies in folate, B-6, and B-12, causing elevated levels in the amino acid homocysteine. Although high levels of homocysteine are conclusively linked to increased risk of cardiovascular disease, scientists are not sure why. High levels of homocysteine appear to reduce the production of nitric oxide in the walls of blood vessels, causing them to become constricted. Also, homocysteine appears to interfere with an anticoagulant protein, possibly contributing to the development of blood clots.

4.
The Heavy Issue of Weight

New clients are often surprised when they come to our clinic for an evaluation of their fitness levels and realize that of all the diagnostics we run, being weighed is not among them. After all, isn't weight one of the important factors in determining who is optimally fit? And isn't it a good idea to establish a baseline, so we'll know when real progress is being made? With regard to fitness, the answer to both questions is no.

When you step on the scale, you're getting a number that reflects a composite of everything inside and out, including your clothing and the breakfast still in your stomach. The variables in the composite render the number nearly meaningless. We always laugh when we're at a fitness center and watch a client stall in front of the demon scale to plead with the instructor, "Couldn't I please take off my shoes before I weigh in?" as if this one divestment will magically reflect true weight loss. We've all heard tales of a creative dieter who tricked the scale into registering fewer pounds by fasting for a day, simmering in a sauna for an hour before the weigh-in, trimming his fingernails, and stripping naked. Of course, after he gets dressed, he celebrates his inevitable weight loss with a drink of water . . . and all the weight is back. Why? Because the guy who just triumphed on the scale was merely naked and dehydrated. He successfully manipulated a number that had no real meaning.

There's no question that being overweight is dangerous to your health. But when we refer to weight, we're really talking about fat. Your training goals do not include losing weight, but they do place high priority on melting fat and getting leaner. Of course, you might lose weight as your program progresses, but don't make that result more important than it is. We're not saying you have to throw away your scale, but from now on, instead of being concerned with how much you weigh, you should be concerned only with how fat you are. In fact, as you get more fit and healthy, build more muscle, lower your fat content, and drop clothing sizes, you might even weigh more than you do right now! Muscle weighs more than fat. Who cares how much you weigh if you're lean, in great shape, and feel wonderful?

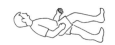

With regard to fitness, the only time you have to be concerned with your actual weight is when your sport has strict weight requirements. Boxing, wrestling, and jockeying come to mind. A word of warning about trying to "make weight" if you think you're too heavy: don't. Doing crazy things like fasting and sweating in a sauna *will* allow the athlete to drop a few pounds, but he or she also runs the risk of cardiac function disturbances, heat stroke, and acutely impaired renal function. Not only is life on the line, but also performance. It takes up to 48 hours to replenish glycogen stores in the muscles, and 24 to 36 hours to recover from dehydration. Frankly, between the final weigh-in and the event, there isn't time to bring the body back to 100 percent. We join the American Medical Association and the American College of Sports Medicine in their condemnation of this practice.

Having launched an assault on weight as a measure of fitness, we will now admit that knowing your weight is useful for four reasons. First, if you're overweight, you're likely carrying too much body fat and are in danger of developing cardiovascular disease. Second, your physician might need to know how much you weigh before prescribing precise dosages of certain medications. Third, you might have to trust equipment that supports your weight, such as a parachute or a bungee cord. And fourth, knowing your weight can provide you with a broad general guideline for comparison to other people of your age, gender, and height. If you discover you're a lot heavier than the table indicates you should be, you'll want to know why, so you can take action to drop fat storage.

To place people in the continuum for comparison, we use the Metropolitan Life Insurance Company Height and Weight Tables. Our experience is that these frequently cited tables offer an intelligent and credible standard. Weights are relevant for people aged twenty-five to fifty-nine. They are based on pounds according to frame and reflect a person dressed in indoor clothing weighing three pounds and shoes with one-inch heels.

WOMEN

HEIGHT (feet/inches)	SMALL FRAME	MEDIUM FRAME	LARGE FRAME
4'10"	102–111	109–121	118–131
4'11"	103–113	111–123	120–134
5'0"	104–115	113–126	122–137
5'1"	106–118	115–129	125–140
5'2"	108–121	118–132	128–143
5'3"	111–124	121–135	131–147
5'4"	114–127	124–138	134–151
5'5"	117–130	127–141	137–155
5'6"	120–133	130–144	140–159
5'7"	123–136	133–147	143–163
5'8"	126–139	136–150	146–167
5'9"	129–142	139–153	149–170
5'10"	132–145	142–156	152–173
5'11"	135–148	145–159	155–176
6'0"	138–151	148–162	158–179

MEN

HEIGHT (feet/inches)	SMALL FRAME	MEDIUM FRAME	LARGE FRAME
5'2"	128–134	131–141	138–150
5'3"	130–136	133–143	140–153
5'4"	132–138	135–145	142–156
5'5"	134–140	137–148	144–160
5'6"	136–142	139–151	146–164
5'7"	138–145	142–154	149–168
5'8"	140–148	145–157	152–172
5'9"	142–151	148–160	155–176
5'10"	144–154	151–163	158–180
5'11"	146–157	154–166	161–184
6'0"	149–160	157–170	164–188
6'1"	152–164	160–174	168–192
6'2"	155–168	164–178	172–197
6'3"	158–172	167–182	176–202
6'4"	162–176	171–187	181–207

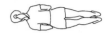

PART TWO

Getting Cardio-Fit

5.
Setting Goals: The Blueprints for Success

One of the ways to make sure you'll be successful in your cardio-fitness program is to have a goal. Starting a program without one is like starting out on a trip without a destination. You would just meander around. You might have a good time, but you'd never know when you had succeeded in getting where you were going. The most successful athletes are those who have a clear sense of outcome: what they want and when they want it. We're going to show you how to set a fitness goal and get there.

If a goal seems like a tall order, you're right. In fact, the prospect of reaching a goal—especially a big one—can seem as overwhelming as unearthing the Holy Grail. After all, a goal is defined as the *final* outcome, with a lot of hard work between now and the moment you reach it. Step up to the challenge! You have nothing to lose and everything to gain.

Before we begin, let's define two terms: "goal" and "objectives." The goal is your final outcome; it's the big picture. Objectives are intermediate benchmarks of progress that line up to get you to your goal. For example, your goal could be to walk one mile without stopping within two months of beginning your program. Your objectives, then, might be to buy good shoes, meet your walking partner for every scheduled workout, be able to walk a quarter of a mile within two weeks, be able to walk half a mile within one month, and be able to walk three quarters of a mile in six weeks. In other words, objectives are stepping stones—small, measurable successes that add up to the big one.

Your goal and objectives will keep you focused on your workout program. Once you're clear about what you want, when you want it, and what you have to do to get it, most decisions and choices in your life will be easier. From now on, when you encounter temptations, you'll ask yourself, "Is this consistent with my goal?" If it's not, it's history. You'll think twice before you dive head-first into a platter of butter cookies if you have a workout in an hour.

SET YOUR GOAL FIRST

The key to setting a fitness goal is to construct a short, simple sentence that states the outcome you expect: what you want and when you want it. Keep it simple and to the point. The goal has to be measurable. For example, you could say, "I run seven miles by my birthday." You can measure that. But you can't say, "I'm strong and fit by my birthday." If you can't quantify "strong and fit," you can't use these words in your goal. Also notice that we construct the goal sentence as if the outcome has already been achieved.

I walk five miles without stopping on May 2.
By Christmas, I swim for forty-five minutes.
My cholesterol level is below 200 by New Year's Eve.

By stating a clear intention (as if the outcome has already been achieved), you set powerful wheels in motion. Before you start your first workout, your body, mind, and spirit are on alert that things have already changed in your life, not the least of which is your attitude. Language is the force that begins the process. In fact, many beginners are able to harness even more incredible focus and discipline by redefining themselves as athletes in their chosen activity. They say, "I am a runner who runs a 10K race on Thanksgiving." There is something transformational about thinking of yourself as an athlete instead of a "normal person" who's pursuing an athletic activity and might feel like an impostor or an outsider. More than once, we've been able to turbocharge a lack-luster fitness program by giving a discouraged jogger a running watch (so he'll look the part) and introducing him to people in our clinic as "Bob, the runner."

No question about it, identity and intention are mystically, yet inarguably, intertwined.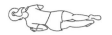

Here's an important tip. When constructing your goal sentence, avoid using words that drain all the power and strength right out of your resolve:

WILL

CAN

TRY

"I WILL walk five miles" means only that the possibility exists somewhere out in the future. The issue of "when" is up for grabs. You might get around to it eventually.

"I CAN walk five miles" means only that you could if you wanted to, but you might not actually do it. It's smug, secretive, and safe.

"I'll TRY to walk five miles" means only that you'll put in some degree of effort, but have no intention of ever doing it. ("I'll try" is a polite brush-off so commonly used in our culture that if you invite someone to join you at a restaurant, and he says, "I'll try," you know he won't show up.)

When we work with an athlete and hear any of these three words, we know we are dealing with a person who has yet to make a commitment to the program and has no confidence. Before the training even begins, our athlete is making excuses for failure. We don't allow this sort of wishy-washy declaration in goal setting. You don't want to either.

OBJECTIVES: STEPS THAT GET THE JOB DONE

Objectives are a series of accomplishments that lead you from your present level of fitness to your goal. One way of understanding the relationship and distinction between the goal and the objectives is to think of the goal as *what* and the objectives as *how*. As we told you earlier, the objectives form a sort of progressive checklist. They can be general: citing a list of accomplishments, the chronology of which will lead you to your goal. Lots of people work backward from the goal to the present moment to design the path. For example, if you want to swim one mile in one month, you'll have to swim three quarters of a mile in three weeks, half a mile in two weeks, and a quarter of a mile in one week; tomorrow you have to book your lane at the pool; today you have to buy a bathing suit; and in an hour you have to get your towel out of the dryer and pack it in your bag. On the other hand, objectives can be very specific—schedules and entries in your log to help keep you on track workout by workout. It's up to you.

PUT IT ALL IN WRITING

As important as it is to state your intentions out loud, writing them down is equally important. Not only will writing help you organize your thoughts, but you'll be able to return to the written page to refresh your memory in the unlikely event that you backslide and wake up one morning with cookie crumbs in your hair, the television remote control clenched in your fist, and three weeks' worth of mail and newspapers on your porch. The enthusiasm and clarity of your original plan will snap you back to reality. Additionally, the written word is a sort of contract with yourself—an agreement that you're serious about getting fit and healthy. In black and white, there's no denying that, at one time, you were on track. Hey! It's *your* handwriting!

WHAT IF I FAIL TO ACHIEVE MY GOAL?

Although we hesitate to address the issue of failure when we're telling you how to succeed, we will be the first to admit that life has an annoying way of broadsiding the best-laid plans. Once you've set your goal, give it your best shot. If you fail, here's how you handle it. On the morning that it's clear that you've failed miserably, set aside five full minutes for shock, denial, guilt, self-loathing, and a wild search for other people to blame. When the five minutes are up, knock it off. It's over.

Setting an amended goal is a matter of understanding what went wrong and then adjusting. Originally, you set either an unrealistic goal, or a realistic goal in an unyielding life. Stuff happened. Circumstances changed. And you got knocked down. So what? Your second goal will be a better one. Don't let failure tempt you to lower the bar to the ground. Keep your sights set high.

Let us tell you the true story of a man who couldn't seem to meet any goals. He attended school only intermittently as he was growing up, but was highly ambitious. As a young man, he threw his hat into the ring for the Illinois General Assembly, but lost the election. So, he enlisted in the military, was assigned to a rifle company, and achieved the rank of captain. Unfortunately, his company disbanded, necessitating his reenlistment as a private. Back to square

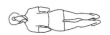

one. After serving in the military, he returned home to work in a store that subsequently went out of business. So he bought a store of his own with a partner. It, too, failed, leaving him badly in debt. His partner died a year later, plunging him further into debt. His sweetheart died the following year. He had a nervous breakdown. After he recovered, he made a bid for the U.S. Congress. He lost the election. He tried again and was elected to the Illinois legislature, but declined the seat in order to run for the U.S. Senate. He lost the election. Then he was nominated to run as the candidate for Republican senator from Illinois, but lost the election after stunning and now famous (and humiliatingly public) debates with his opponent. What a loser! Right? Wrong. This man who couldn't seem to achieve any goal was Abraham Lincoln. As you know, in 1860 he was elected the sixteenth president and the first Republican. And his list of accomplishments is etched in our history as among the most important and significant made by any leader. The point is that failure is a teacher. You set a new goal and go on with your life.

Do you have to wait until you're in full-blown failure before you adjust your goal? No. Don't be so rigid that you can't recognize when circumstances have changed and scooted your goal just out of reach. In fact, we would be willing to wager that most injuries occur in sports when an athlete is so fixated on the goal that he or she competes with an injury or illness, on a day when the playing conditions are dangerous, or when equipment isn't quite right. There's a fine line between passion for your sport and blind obsession. Don't cross it.

FINAL WORD

Can you have more than one goal? Certainly. But we urge you to keep it all simple. One well-chosen goal can change your whole life.

6.
No More Excuses

For every fitness program that stalls, there are a thousand excuses. For every program that never gets off the ground, there are even more. In fact, designing a fitness regimen for a new client has become a two-step process. First we put together the program. Easy. And then we hurdle all the excuses. Hard. Over the years, we've heard every excuse for missing a workout ever concocted by a fidgeting new athlete with a dry mouth who can't make eye contact. Needless to say, some are more imaginative than others. (Our personal favorite involved planets in a particularly ominous alignment with something insidious in retrograde. We won't bore you with details. Trust us. We could hardly keep straight faces.) Of all the excuses we hear (from the ridiculous to the legitimate), there is *one* recurring excuse that crops up at the outset of nearly every program: "I don't have time."

If you think you don't have time, you're mistaken. You do. Here's the solution to your dilemma: stop trying to make time to work out. You can't *make* time. It is a finite commodity in your busy life: only twenty-four hours every day. No more. Although you can't make time, you can *take* it. Simple truth. For everything new you add to your schedule, you have to give something up. But what?

Take a pad and keep a detailed log for a couple of days. If you're like most of us, the scheduled, non-negotiable events of your day will look something like this:

Wake up, shower, dress, eat breakfast—one hour

Commute to office—thirty minutes

Work—nine hours (with a quick lunch sneaked in)

Commute home—thirty minutes

Dinner with family—thirty minutes

Sleep—eight hours

Wow! This looks like a pretty crammed day, doesn't it? But take out your calculator, and you'll notice that if you add up all the scheduled, non-negotiable events, they total nineteen hours and thirty minutes. Last time we looked, there were twenty-four hours in a day. That means you've got four hours and thirty minutes *every* day when you're apparently not doing anything special. That's a total of twenty-two hours and thirty minutes during the work week. And we haven't even added in weekends yet. There are another forty-eight hours! By our calculations, you could swing by the track three times a week for an hour each time and *still* have more than forty-five hours left over. Right?

Okay. Maybe we're being too simplistic. But you get the message. You *do* have the time. You're just using it for activities other than working out. Simply figure out what you're doing during those forty-five or so hours every week, and decide what you would be willing to give up in exchange for having fun, enjoying good health, feeling wonderful, and looking great. Our bet is that whatever you sacrifice will have been of no real consequence.

One embellishment to the excuse "I don't have the time" is "I'm so hammered at work, I have to rest in my spare time." We've got news for you. If you're so hammered at work that you have no energy left for a workout, you need to work out. It's not as crazy as it sounds. Working out gives you energy and stamina to fully enjoy the other facets of your life. As for getting rest, fear not. You sleep much better when you're physically active. Before you know it, you'll wonder how you ever managed to be so entertained and fulfilled by a recliner and a TV with cable. (By the way, let us take this opportunity to remark that although a TV program can be quite exciting, and can get your heart racing, this in no way constitutes a cardio-fitness workout. Sorry.)

If you think of time spent working out as lost time, think again. Researchers tell us that engaging in a regular exercise program such as the ones listed in this book can prolong your life by years. Not only will you have *more* time in your life, but the time you have will be high quality. Working out is an investment of time that yields generous dividends.

GETTING THE SCHEDULE TOGETHER

Once you've decided when you're going to train, log those workouts into your daily planner in ink as if they were business appointments. Now, to be honest, keeping your workout appointments will be difficult at first. We know beginners who think of the workout as "play," and regard taking time to train as capricious. They are racked by guilt that leaves the appointment vulnerable to any "responsible" task that elbows its way up to that time slot. Worse, employers and coworkers who see "In-line skating 5:30" on the Tuesday schedule will be less than thrilled when an aspiring athlete hesitates to stay after work to discuss a last-minute change in a contract. For this reason, we suggest that you begin your new program with little white lies in your calendar: entries that carry a little more weight for you and anyone with prying eyes. Develop a code. One of our clients enters into her calendar "Board meeting 5:30." No one at work realizes her meeting is with a *snow*board. But coworkers have noticed that she's more focused and alert in the office, and probably assume that her position on the board is giving her a huge professional boost. Our lips are sealed. We won't tell if you won't.

TEN WAYS TO BEAT AN EXCUSE

There are times when it's necessary to scrap a scheduled workout. But for every one of us, there comes a day when a workout is simply too much of a hassle. You know you should head out the door, but you just don't feel like it. Don't cave in. There's more at stake than just the workout. Working out when you don't really want to is one of the ways you'll develop the will and discipline of a champion athlete. When you're tempted to skip a workout for no good reason, and you find yourself inventing outrageous reasons to justify your newfound sloth, here are ten effective ways to beat those lame excuses and get yourself out the door:

1. *Review your written goal and objectives.* Think of them as promises you made to yourself to regain control over your life, and ask yourself if the payoff for missing your workout will be greater than the benefit you'll receive if you go ahead and work out. The answer likely will be NO. Out the door you go.

2. *Don't think about the whole workout if it's overwhelming you.* Just get dressed, pack your workout bag, and step out the front door. All athletes will confide that this is often the hardest part of the workout. Once you're out the front door, you've already won the battle.

3. *Delay the workout.* Don't be tempted to cancel a workout when all you really need to do is reschedule it to accommodate a conflict. Consider the delay an IOU on which you'll collect in a few hours. Better late than never.

4. *Break the workout into halves.* If you can't squeeze in a complete workout, go ahead and do as much as you can. You can finish the workout later. Researchers tell us that two thirty-minute workouts can be as effective as a single one-hour workout. In fact, you might even enjoy a little kick-start in the morning followed by a stress buster at the end of the day. Just remember that each segment should be at least thirty minutes of sustained effort for you to get a cardiovascular benefit.

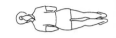

5. *Keep a log.* There's nothing more satisfying than filling the pages of a training log with records of successful workouts, and there's nothing more abysmal than a black hole in the middle of a full page. There's a lot to be said for the momentum of a streak of successes that you won't want to break.

6. *Work out with a friend.* Many a lame excuse has been dealt a death blow by an athlete with good manners and a sense of loyalty to a cranky friend waiting in the dark and cold at the track.

7. *Make a mental list of all the reasons you deserve to be healthy, happy, lean, strong, and in control.* Then go out and seize the day.

8. *Rely on momentum.* Once you're already in motion, keep it going. For example, tag a workout onto the end of an active day. Work out right after you leave the office in the evening, before you head home and get too relaxed.

9. *Remember that working out is fun.* Actually, it's unfortunate that we call training "*working* out," because the connotations of the word "working" are those of duty, difficulty, responsibility, and obligation. In reality, training is joyful and exciting. No matter how tough it is to get to your workout, once you're there, you'll have a ball. Guaranteed.

10. *Set your training schedule and make the decision once to keep it on track.* Don't force yourself to remake that same decision every day or you'll find yourself in conflict over and over and over.

No more excuses. Now, get going!

7.
How to Know When You're Working Out Hard Enough, and When You're Not

It's important to exercise at the proper intensity. If you work out too hard, you'll get exhausted, discouraged, and injured. If you don't work out hard enough, you'll fail to see results, decide that the program is a huge waste of your time, and abandon the workout. One of the easiest ways to gauge the level of your intensity is with the Rate of Perceived Exertion (RPE). Very simply, it's gauging intensity by asking a basic question: "How do I *feel?*" Sitting stock-still in an easy chair will have a rating of 0. Walking at a brisk pace, where you can still talk and haven't thought of throwing up yet, is a 3. Doing something really strenuous, like pushing your car up a hill, is a 9 or 10. For results in cardiovascular training found in these programs, you want to be working out at an RPE between 3 and 5.

THE RPE SCALE

0	—no exertion
1	—very weak
2	—weak
3	—moderate
4	—somewhat strong
5	—strong
6	—stronger
7	—very strong
8	—very, very strong
9	—extremely strong
10	—maximum exertion, uncomfortable

NOT ALL ACTIVITIES ARE CREATED EQUAL: HOW TO TELL

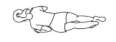

It goes without saying that running is more strenuous than walking, but some distinctions are not so obvious. When you're trying to select an activity that gets your heart rate up, it's important to know which one will do the job so you'll get maximum benefit for your time and effort. It's also interesting to know which activities are equal to the one you've selected, just in case you decide to switch. Measuring "equivalency" in terms of effort was developed for injured athletes who needed to keep fitness levels high while they recovered. For example, if a sprinter breaks a bone in her foot and has to lay off for a little while, she can turn to swimming or cycling—activities that will get her heart rate up without putting strain on the broken foot. This way, she can keep her cardiovascular conditioning at a high level until she can return to the track. In determining which sports can create this crossover, scientists have developed a simple rating system to quantify effort. Now, if you want to switch, it's easy to find a sport that will require the same effort. Or if you choose a new sport that requires more or less effort than the training you now use, you'll know how to adjust the new workout to get the benefit you're used to.

Because the goal of endurance exercise is to get the heart rate up, scientists measure the amount of oxygen consumed in one minute. This is called metabolic equivalent, or MET. Scientists start with a baseline: the amount of energy you expend when you're sitting still. This MET level is designated as 1. If you do something that burns three times as much energy as sitting still, the MET level will be 3. You get the picture. While it can be argued that not everyone expends the same amount of energy in each activity, the MET level isn't designed to measure precise effort; it's designed to give you a basis for general comparison. For example, if you enjoy waterskiing (MET level 6.8) and want an equal activity, you might choose snowboarding (MET level 6.8) or hill climbing (MET level 6.8) without a pack. If you run (MET level 10.2), you know that you'll have to cycle for about three minutes (MET level 3.5) to equal the benefits of one minute of running.

USING YOUR HEART RATE AS A GUIDE TO YOUR WORKOUT

In coaching and supervising workouts, we like to train people depending on how they feel. We suggest you learn to rely on self-assessment and good judgment. If you're feeling strained and winded, back off. If you're feeling great, go for it. But if you would like to be more precise, there are simple, accepted guidelines that will give you a general idea of how you're doing from your

MET VALUE TABLE

ACTIVITY	MET VALUE
Bicycling: leisure	4
Bicycling: 10–11.9 mph, light	6
Bicycling: 12–13.9 mph, moderate	8
Bicycling: 14–15.9 mph, vigorous	10
Bicycling: 16–19 mph, racing	12
Bicycling: > 20 mph, racing	16
Stationary bicycling: very light	3
Stationary bicycling: light	5.5
Stationary bicycling: moderate	7
Stationary bicycling: vigorous	10.5
Stationary bicycling: very vigorous	12.5
Circuit resistance training	8
Resistance training: light	3
Resistance training: vigorous	6
Stretching, yoga	4
Water aerobics	4
Aerobics: general	6
Aerobics: low impact	5
Aerobics: high impact	7
Jogging: general	7
Running: 5 mph (12 min. mile)	8
Running: 5.2 mph (11.5 min. mile)	9
Running: 6 mph (10 min. mile)	10
Running: 6.7 mph (9 min. mile)	11
Running: 7 mph (8.5 min. mile)	11.5
Running: 7.5 mph (8 min. mile)	12.5
Running: 8 mph (7.5 min. mile)	13.5
Running: 8.6 mph (7 min. mile)	14
Running: 9 mph (6.5 min. mile)	15
Running: 10 mph (6 min. mile)	16
Running: 10.9 mph (5.5 min. mile)	18
Running: cross-country	9
Running: up stairs	15

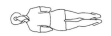

ACTIVITY	MET VALUE
Golf: general	4.5
Golf: carrying clubs	5.5
Golf: pulling clubs	5
Golf: using power cart	3.5
Tennis: practice	7
Tennis: doubles	6
Tennis: singles	8
Walking: < 2.0 mph, very slow	2
Walking: 2.0 mph, slow	2.5
Walking: 2.5 mph	3
Walking: 3.0 mph, moderate	3.5
Walking: 3.5 mph, brisk	4
Walking uphill: 3.5 mph	6
Walking: 4.0 mph, very brisk	4
Walking: 4.5 mph, very, very brisk	4.5
Walking: for pleasure, with the dog	3.5
Walking: to work or class	4
Swimming: laps-freestyle, vigorous	10
Swimming: laps-freestyle, light/moderate	8
Swimming: backstroke, general	8
Swimming: breaststroke, general	10
Swimming: butterfly, general	11
Swimming: leisurely, not laps	6
Swimming: sidestroke, general	8
Skiing: general	7
Skiing: cross-country, light effort	7
Skiing: cross-country, moderate effort	8
Skiing: cross-country, vigorous effort	14
Skiing: downhill, light effort	5
Skiing: downhill, moderate effort	6
Skiing: downhill, vigorous effort	8
Calisthenics: pushups, situps, vigorous	8
Calisthenics: light/moderate, back exercises	4.5

heart's point of view. We do this by determining minimum and maximum target heart rates defined in beats per minute. (Don't panic yourself by considering the possibilities of that moment just beyond the maximum target heart rate. Exceeding the max will not result in instant death.) These numbers are general guidelines based on your age. Get out your calculator. To determine your target heart rate, subtract your age from 220. Multiply that number by 50 percent (.50) to determine your minimum target heart rate. Multiply that same number by 75 percent (.75) to determine your maximum target heart rate. Your goal should be to stay within the range between minimum and maximum. Simply put, if you're out for an easy workout, work closer to the minimum. If you're out to pour it on, work closer to the maximum. If you are 35 years old:

$$
\begin{array}{cc}
220 & 220 \\
-35 & -35 \\
\hline
185 & 185 \\
\times.50 & \times.75 \\
\hline
\text{92.50 minimum heart rate} & \text{128.75 maximum heart rate}
\end{array}
$$

Although we use the general terms in your schedule for expressing effort and pace, we're really talking about your target heart rate. Exceeding your maximum target heart rate might mean that you're working far too hard and need to drop back. On the other hand, if you can't even hit the minimum of your target heart rate in your workout, you might not be working hard enough and might need to step up your pace a bit (as long as everything else is working well and your body is conditioned to handle the increased load).

To interpret your effort, determine your target heart rate. If you're at the low end of the range, you're working easily. If you're in the middle, you're working moderately. If you're near the high end, you're working hard. It's a simple principle.

Even if you never bother to calculate your target heart rate, learn to read your body's signals, use your own judgment, and rely heavily on your answer to the question "How do I feel?"

HOW TO TAKE YOUR PULSE

If you want a quick check of what your heart is doing, check your pulse to count heartbeats per minute. No need to carry a stethoscope or a heart monitor

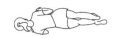

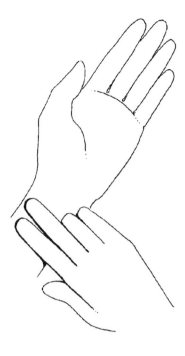

to check your own pulse. Nature has provided us with two wonderful checkpoints: one on your wrist and one on your throat. All you need is two fingertips and a watch that ticks off seconds.

Wrist

Place your index and middle fingertips of your right hand between your wrist bone and the tendon on the thumb side of your left wrist (palm up). How will you know you have the right spot and you're exerting enough pressure? Simple. You'll feel the pulse distinctly but won't be uncomfortable. Another important tip is to stop exercising or moving when you take your pulse. Jostling isn't helpful.

Throat

Place your index and middle fingertips of your right hand along the left side of your neck just to the rear of your windpipe. Gently move and press with your

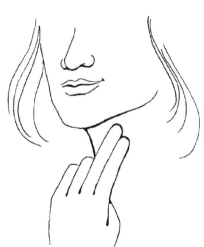

fingertips until you locate the pulse. Keep the pressure gentle. Too much pressure will depress the artery you've just located and block the flow. Again, stop moving and be still when you take your pulse.

Count

No matter how good (or not) you are at math, the count is simple. Many people find it best to start the count when the second hand (or the digital readout) of the watch is at 12. When the moment is right, start counting beats. If you're a whiz at math, count beats for ten seconds and multiply by six. If you're pretty good, count beats for fifteen seconds and multiply by four. If math wasn't your best subject at all, count for thirty seconds and multiply by two. If you're really shaky around numbers, just count for the entire minute.

INTERPRETING THE NUMBERS

AGE	TARGET HEART RATE (BEATS PER MINUTE) MIN AND MAX
15	103–154
20	100–150
25	98–146
30	95–143
35	93–139
40	90–135
45	88–131
50	85–128
55	83–124
60	80–120
65	78–116
70	75–113
75	73–109

PRECISION NUMBERS WITH A FLICK OF YOUR WRIST: A HEART-RATE MONITOR

After a track workout a few years ago, our running buddy's young son invited us to join him as he watched a *Star Trek* episode on television. At the point we tuned in, there had been some sort of intergalactic battle between the *Enterprise* and an evil alien warship. The aliens must have been kicking some serious booty, because the *Enterprise* sick bay was wall to wall with bloodied Federation crew members. The little boy was riveted to the television as the starship's physician raced from patient to patient, attaching tiny transmitters that monitored life signs and telegraphed them to screens over each table. At the first commercial, the kid turned to us and whispered, "Isn't this cool? Don't you wish the future was now?" Phil laughed and said, "In some ways, it is!" He

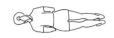

lifted his sweatshirt, revealing a slender black strap wrapped around his chest. "This is the monitor I use for reading my heart rate when I run. The numbers are transmitted to this 'watch' on my wrist." The kid was more than impressed.

When you train, it's important to know how hard you're working. You can do this a couple of ways. One way is to stop occasionally and take your pulse. The other is to wear a heart-rate monitor. Today, heart-rate monitors are small, inexpensive, battery-operated biofeedback devices that give you accurate readings of your heart rate. They work similarly to the electrocardiograph (ECG) you'll find in a cardiologist's office. Basically, the technology relies on two electrodes mounted on a belt that you strap around your chest or that are imbedded in the inside seam of a sports bra. The electrodes pick up the electrical impulses from your heart and relay that data to the receiver on your wrist. A quick glance at your wrist gives you all the information you need to know how hard your heart is working. Almost all monitors can be programmed to settings you determine to be the upper and lower limits of your target heart rate. As you near one of those limits, the monitor will alert you with a beep to let you know when to slow down or speed up. Many manufacturers have customized the receiver to snap onto the handlebars of a bike, or fit into a harness for a swimmer, or attach to a piece of gym equipment. More advanced monitors are designed to be used in conjunction with your computer. You can download your data—heart rate and times—directly to your electronic training log to keep accurate records that can help you spot progress or problems and make adjustments.

You need to make two decisions before you go shopping for a monitor. First, what do you want it to do? And second, how much are you willing to spend? In exploring heart-rate monitors, talk to friends who've used them; they're a great resource for information. They aren't out to sell you anything, so they'll tell you the truth about their monitors: what they like and what they don't. If you're lucky, they'll even let you try it out. Then, hit the Internet for companies that retail monitors. Be sure you're looking at personal heart-rate monitors designed for athletes, and not hospital equipment (unless you have a million-dollar budget and are willing to drag a crash cart around the track). You'll find companies all over the world that will sell directly to you, and some that will refer you to distributors in your area. Shop carefully. Deal only with a company that will stand behind its monitor with a money-back guarantee, a comprehensive warranty, and the ability to repair or replace rapidly . . . just in case. Additionally, ask the company to send you an instruction book for operating the monitor and designing programs with it. The more you know about the features and capabilities of your new monitor, the more useful it will be.

A quick word about heart-rate monitor etiquette: turn off the sound on your monitor when you're working out with other people. If you set your monitor to beep constantly in rhythm to your heartbeat, you'll throw off the cadence of other people, and seriously annoy them. Silence the alarm too. If an alarm goes off on your wrist, our high-tech culture has conditioned us to react immediately: figure out what's beeping, why it's beeping, and what we must do to stop it. You don't want to break the concentration of other athletes. It could turn ugly. We heard a story about a guy who made the mistake of wearing a heart-rate monitor during the New York City Marathon a couple of years ago. As the tale is told, he had set his monitor to beep with every beat of his heart. Although the constant *beep-beep-beep-beep* might have set an entertaining pace for him, mile after mile it was driving the runners around him insane. Reportedly, they kept stumbling, unable to settle into their own rhythms. They begged him to silence the beeping monitor, but he refused to comply. When the pack could stand this guy no longer, they cornered him against a railing on the 59th Street Bridge at the fifteen-mile mark, removed his wrist receiver, and unceremoniously tossed it into the river. He's lucky that's all they tossed. We're not saying the runners who de-beeped this guy were right. We're not even telling you the tale is true. We're just warning you that not everyone will be as fascinated by your heart rate as you are. Be courteous.

8.
Red Lights: Signals That You Need to Back Off a Workout or Quit

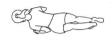

Before you begin any exercise program, you *must* consult your physician to be certain that the workout is safe for you. Once you've been cleared to begin your training, you'll need to follow the simple, commonsense guidelines for exercising developed by our good friend, the late Dr. Michael Pollock, the world-renowned researcher and exercise physiologist from the University of Florida Department of Human Performance.

1. Exercise only when you feel well.

2. If you're planning a no-holds-barred workout, wait a couple of hours after eating.

3. Adjust your workout to suit the weather and time of day.

4. Wear proper clothing and shoes. Use the right equipment.

5. Know your limitations and get your physician's okay.

6. Start slowly and progress gradually.

FIVE RED LIGHTS: SYMPTOMS THAT MEAN STOP YOUR WORKOUT!

In the course of your workout, you need to constantly monitor your body for signals that tell you what's working properly and what's not. Phil compares this monitoring to sitting in the cockpit of a jet fighter. He says that when he's running, he imagines a sort of control panel in front of his face. On it are dozens of gauges, dials, and meters that he adjusts to achieve maximum workout performance. A little more speed here. A little more pressure there. Pour it on. Back it off. Throttle forward. Throttle back. As in Phil's imaginary cockpit, your body provides you with feedback. Among them are warning lights that flash on and let you know you're in trouble. They are signals that you must cease your workout immediately, without hesitation.

1. *Discomfort in any degree of severity in the upper body: chest, arms, neck, and jaw.*

The symptoms of a heart attack have been described as an ache, burn, tightness, pressure, or sensation of fullness. The sensation can be subtle. It shouldn't have to drop you to your knees to get your attention. Forgo the old "this can't be happening to me" routine. It is. Dial 911 for an ambulance, take an aspirin (no kidding), and lie down. Right now. Sure, it could be heartburn, but it could also be a heart attack. Early intervention saves lives. Don't take chances.

2. *Faintness, light-headedness, or nausea.*

No matter how fleeting the moment, feeling faint or light-headed should signal you to take a time-out and reassess the situation. While it's true that you might be experiencing the result of having skipped breakfast, it's also possible that you're suffering from something far more serious. At best, you might be moments away from embarrassing yourself and scaring the wits out of your workout partner by sliding face first onto the floor. At worst, you might be receiving an important signal your body is sending regarding diminished blood flow. Even if it goes away, you need to tell your physician about it as soon as possible.

3. *Shortness of breath, effort, wheezing, or inability to recover to easy breathing within five minutes.*

We can't tell you how many times we've seen someone try to laugh this one off with a self-deprecating "Whooooa! I'm outta shape!" While it's true that being out of shape can tax the cardiovascular system in a workout harder than you're used to, it can also signal serious problems. We regard the ability to breathe as crucial to life as we know it. If you're experiencing difficulty, take a break. Get your body to settle down. Pay particular attention if you discover yourself using ancillary muscles to force air into your lungs; for example, if you're unconsciously lifting your shoulders to try to increase lung capacity. If, after five minutes of rest, you can't pull yourself together, dial 911 for an ambulance, take an aspirin, and lie down.

4. *Discomfort or pain in bones or joints during or after exercise.*

Fitness comes through a series of adaptations. You apply a measured amount of stress, and the body adapts to it and becomes stronger in a gradual cycle of breaking down and building up. We have to be honest with you. There *is* discomfort in the breaking-down phase, right before adapting and building. But well-trained athletes always describe this discomfort as a "good" ache. Notice that we have not used the word "pain." Nothing should

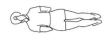

hurt you to the point of pain. You have to pay attention to your body. Expect muscle aches and slight discomfort as you push yourself from level to level, but *never* accept pain in bones and joints. If you have pain in bones and joints, you might be headed for serious and possibly permanent injuries of bones, soft tissues, tendons, and ligaments. A trip to a physiatrist for testing and treatment might help you get control of an underlying injury and prevent future problems. By the way, your bones do participate in the cycle of breaking down and building up. This is the reason that load-bearing exercise is recommended for mitigating the bone-diminishing effects of osteoporosis. But again, bones and joints should not hurt.

5. *Unspecified pain.*

At no time should an exercise hurt. There's no doubt that sometimes a workout can be challenging and uncomfortable. Discomfort is your body's way of telling you that you're working hard. But pain has another message. Pain is your body's way of identifying a point of injury and instantaneously activating your entire system to wrench you away from the stressor to protect you from further harm. If you allow an exercise to hurt, you're going to have to override your body's natural instincts to protect itself, which isn't easy. Your muscles tighten as they get ready to take flight but are not allowed to. Working out a specific muscle when all those around it are firing to deal with pain makes the workout ineffective. More important, it's not smart. Your body is trying to tell you something. Pain is injury. Back off.

TEN WARNING SIGNS THAT IT'S TIME TO TAKE TIME OFF

There comes a time when the body demands rest. You know that time has come when you notice signs of overtraining. It's time to take some time off when:

1. *You can't finish a workout you easily completed two days ago.*

Every athlete experiences one magical moment in training when all the pieces come together and the workout is effortless. Phil calls this reaching "Air Velvet" in running. No time. No space. No work. No contact with the earth. Just free flow. Having experienced it once, you'll probably try to get into that effortless space again. Not to disappoint you, but the magic doesn't come often. So you'll likely be disappointed as much as you are inspired. If you can't get into Air Velvet again right away, don't worry. It'll come. But that's not what we're talking about. We're talking about a marked deterioration of your workout, whether or not the last one required effort. If you could walk a mile on Monday, you should be able to walk that same mile—and probably a little more—on Wednesday. If you can't, then something's wrong. Your body might be tired and not ready to resume hard effort.

2. *Yesterday you were yakking up a storm and today, in the exact same workout, you're unable to speak in full sentences.*

Grunting in response to your partner's remarks doesn't count. Neither does whining. If you are unable to hit a comfortable pace, even though you did so in your last workout (which was identical), back off.

3. *You feel "icky" before, during, or after the workout.*

We warned you about several potentially serious symptoms during and after your workout. But we want to extend the scope. Overtrained athletes complain of feeling icky: it's a case of the blahs and the feeling that something's wrong, even though you might not be able to identify the source of your problem. The ick creeps up on you and hangs over every facet of your life like a wet blanket.

4. *You feel tired all the time.*

You fall asleep standing up and drool down the front of your shirt (not attractive and certainly annoying to your coworkers). And your family notices a certain reluctance on your part to participate in normal daily routines, like getting your clothes off before you step into the shower. Give your body a rest.

5. *You can't sleep.*

This is by far one of the most confusing, ironic symptoms of overtraining. You're exhausted, yet you toss and turn all night. Go figure. And when you do manage to finally fall asleep, you can be certain that it'll be a short, disturbed snooze. (This, of course, will exhaust your spouse, who will begin to exhibit signs of overtraining without having to train. Can you deal with guilt?)

6. *You have generalized aches and pains.*

Aches and pains demand close scrutiny. They might alert you that you're overtraining, and will go away with a little layoff. But if they're signaling an injury, this is one symptom that laying off might not mitigate. Pay attention and make good decisions that will not have long-term consequences.

7. *Your pulse is elevated in the morning before you even move.*

When you first begin aerobic training, you might become obsessed with getting the old heart rate up. But not before you get out of bed. Get familiar with your resting pulse. If you're not feeling right in the morning, take your pulse. If it's elevated by even a few beats, you need to consider scrapping your workouts for a day or so.

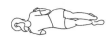

8. *You are irritable.*

For some of us, irritability is a natural and constant state of being, but if you're a good-natured person who suddenly morphs into the Antichrist, look no farther than your training log. Back off until you're back to your old sweet self. And, as an apology, make copies of your training log for everyone you trashed before you discovered the problem and solution. Not only will this stand up as evidence of temporary insanity, but it will certainly impress your friends and family.

9. *You are suddenly susceptible to every cold on the planet.*

Let us assure you that the cold in your head is not "all in your head." It's very real. Athletes who are overtrained are worn down and worn out. This makes them vulnerable to communicable illnesses. The common cold seems to be the poster child for this phenomenon. You have only to observe marathon runners in the weeks before their marathon. Among their other rituals and prerace practices, they avoid crowds. Why? They recognize that they're on that edge of being overtrained. If there's an illness out there that requires sprays and tissues, it'll be attracted to them like a heat-seeking missile. No need to regard every sniffle as a sure sign that you've overdone your training; it's probably just a little warning. Of course, two colds in one season . . . ah, that's another matter.

10. *You dread your workout.*

It's natural for you to experience a little anxiety or annoyance before the intrusion of a workout into your busy schedule. We'll be the first to admit that it's simple to come up with good excuses for skipping a workout. But it's just as simple to come up with compelling reasons you need to get off your duff and out the door. It's a private debate that beginners wage on a regular basis. To sweat or not to sweat? That is the question. Go ahead and ponder the two options. If you choose to skip two workouts in a row, something is very wrong—especially if you were having fun right up until the moment when you could no longer take your workout clothes out of the dryer without clenching your teeth, squinting your eyes, and moaning softly. You need to consider the possibility that you're overtrained and your body is commanding you to back off.

WHAT IF I HAVE TO MISS A WORKOUT IN MY TRAINING SCHEDULE?

You'll live. Quickly figure out what happened and what you'll have to do to keep it from happening again. First, we want you back on the training schedule as soon as possible, before you decide that you actually like being idle. And second, we don't want you to lose any of your hard-earned conditioning. Don't waste time and energy on guilt. It's a useless emotion that masks the fact that you made a choice. You had your reason. A good reason for missing a workout would be something like recovering from a small injury. A bad reason for missing a workout would be something like a cowboy-movie marathon on your favorite cable station. No matter what the reason, as easily as you chose to miss the workout, you can choose to return to your training. Just get back on your schedule as soon as possible.

Here are general guidelines for resuming your training schedule after a layoff. If you follow our suggestion and still don't feel right, continue to back up until you find a workout that's comfortable. Start there. At no point should you push it or you'll end up injured (and having to watch even more cowboy-movie marathons in traction on the couch).

If you miss one to two days, ignore it and pick up the schedule where you left off.

If you miss three days, back up the schedule one day.

If you miss four days, back up the schedule two days.

If you miss five days, back up the schedule three days.

If you miss six days, back up the schedule four days.

If you miss seven days to two weeks, repeat the last full week you did before you suspended training, but cut it in half. Then repeat it again with a full schedule. Now resume training.

If you miss three weeks, repeat the last week you did before you suspended training, but cut it in half. Then repeat it again, but cut it to three quarters. Then repeat it again with a full schedule. Now resume normal training.

If you miss more than three weeks but fewer than six, go back to the beginning of the phase you're in and start over. If you suspended the schedule less than halfway through a phase, back all the way up to the beginning of the previous phase.

If you miss more than six weeks, go back to the beginning of the whole schedule and start over. Don't waste time on despair. Just get back into action.

IS THERE A "BETTER" TIME OF DAY TO WORK OUT?

Yep, whenever you can. We once organized a training schedule for a friend whose physician had suggested running as a stress buster. The prescription for running shoes came in the nick of time, because our friend was a hard-driven executive with a killer schedule who described herself as a "woman on the edge." It was true. She was suffering from hypertension and tension headaches with the certain promise that more medical problems were right around the corner. Putting together a beginning program for her was a privilege, and easy to do. Once we knew what we were going to do, we came to the issue of "when." After examining her 9-pound day planner, consulting her administrative assistant, and downloading her Palm Pilot, we found that her only uncommitted time was at dawn. We suggested that she get up thirty minutes early three days a week, and come to the track where we would work her out. We thought she would be so pleased and impressed with our creative time management. Instead she pointed out the obvious: when she was asleep, it was the *only* time she was *not* stressed out, and that if we hauled her out of bed before the dawn's early light, she would be even *more* stressed out, so *get real, Whartons!!!* We all had a good laugh. And found another time slot.

In defense of dawn, some athletes enjoy working out first thing in the morning to get their bodies moving and awake. This gets the workout out of the way before life broadsides a busy schedule like our friend's. (However, you must promise not to show up for work so pleased with yourself that you become smug and obnoxious in the eyes of your fellow coworkers who couldn't even get their hair combed.) On the other hand, some people feel too sluggish in the morning to get anything moving. They can barely manage to lift a coffee cup and are just glad if they can knock it over and lap up the coffee off the kitchen table. In their defense, some studies suggest that leaping out of bed and throwing oneself into immediate exertion might put strain on a body that's not warmed up and a heart that's not ready to pound yet. If you choose to work out at dawn, take an extra few minutes to warm up and get your juices flowing before you begin. You might enjoy working out at the end of the day to release stress and tension. Or you might be able to sneak off in the middle of the day for a workout. This strategy works only if you have access to a shower and a changing room, and can grab a bite to eat on your way back to the job. Under no circumstances are you to skip a meal in order to work out. Another favorite time to work out when schedules are generally merciful is right before bed. Contrary to conventional wisdom, working out before bedtime is not necessarily a dreaded insomnia producer. We do it all the time. We simply allow about thirty minutes between the workout and bedtime to cool down, stretch, shower, make sure we've had plenty of water, toss our workout clothes in the hamper, and settle down as relaxation settles in. A great surprise benefit of working out—no matter what time—is that you tire your body physically, so your sleep will improve.

PART THREE

Getting Started

9.
Putting Your Cardio-Fitness Program Together

This section of the book is a catalog of ten activities that provide superior cardiovascular workouts that we have selected from many possibilities. We'll tell you a few things about technique, what to wear, what equipment you'll need, and what the sports medicine specialists warn us about the activity and its potential for injury. We'll also give you a few tips from experts who coach athletes in the following activities:

Walking
Racewalking
Running
Jumping rope
Dancing
Swimming
In-line skating

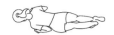

Cross-country skiing

Cycling

Rowing

All you have to do is choose your favorite activity and flip to the training schedule, where you'll find a year of workouts just for you!

THE PATTERN OF YOUR TRAINING SCHEDULE

You'll notice that we've organized a full year of training day by day for you and have divided it into phases: beginner, intermediate, and advanced. Within each distinct phase are four levels of development:

1. Awakening the body. Here we gently introduce your body to increased load, putting all systems on alert so they can begin to make slow adjustments to new demands.

2. Laying the foundation. There's nothing that causes an injury or a shutdown faster than doing too much too soon, so we lay in a foundation of skill and pattern that your muscles and cardiovascular system can handle before we really start to work.

3. Building endurance. Once the body is prepared, we increase the cardiovascular demand so your heart can work a little harder and get stronger.

4. Achieving mastery. At the end of each phase, you'll have achieved the goals of that cycle and be ready for more.

The workouts are designed on the unique cycles of nature: hard and easy workouts within hard and easy weeks within hard and easy months. You'll be able to train hard and recover quickly without injury.

THUMBS UP ON TEACHING YOU THE ACTIVITY

It's impossible for us to teach you all you'll need to know about your activity in the few pages of the section we've devoted to it. We are going to assume that you already know at least a little about the activity you've selected. If you don't know how to handle the activity, get in touch with a good teacher or coach, or join a class.

The best we can do is to illustrate the activity with an animation that will give you some idea about proper technique. To see the animation, flip the pages of the book with your thumb and look into the margins. You'll see a team of little athletes as they demonstrate technique up and down the edge of the pages. We call this our "thumb-cathalon" . . . ten athletic events that you can trigger with your thumb.

WHAT'S A GAME DAY?

In the advanced phase of each sport, we've inserted Game Days. Because we believe that training is a means rather than an end, we reward you with days when you'll go out and enjoy your fit, lean body. On Game Day, you can play another sport, or engage in another physical activity—anything, as long as you have a great time and start to realize the potential of the body you've created.

WHEN WE TALK ABOUT EFFORT OR PACE

Let's review the concept of effort and your target heart rate. Use a heart-rate monitor or take your pulse at rest to determine your target heart-rate range: from minimum to maximum. At any given moment in a workout, you can interpret your effort by your heart rate. If you're at the low end of the range, you're working easily. If you're in the middle, you're working moderately. If you're near the high end, you're working hard. It's a simple principle.

Even if you never bother to calculate your target heart rate, remember to read your body's signals, use your own judgment, and rely heavily on your answer to the question *"How do I feel?"*

THE CARDIO-FITNESS PROGRAM YOU'VE SELECTED IS GREAT, BUT IT'S NOT PERFECT

We have to admit that although any of these activities is a great cardio-fitness program, it's not the perfect workout. Fitness has several components: strength, flexibility, health, and stamina. You've got stamina handled. But you're going to need to consider supplementing your program with flexibility and strength work. (We happen to know two great guys who wrote two great books on the subject—what were the chances?)

On the second, fourth, and sixth days of each week of your training, we remind you on your schedule that you need to do some strength work not just to help your workouts, but to take up the slack on muscles that are not used, or are not used enough, within the narrow requirements of your activity. And we're counting on you to take the time.

We also advise you to put together a flexibility program for several reasons: you need flexibility so your joints will be able to go through their full ranges of motion. Stretching helps your muscles flush metabolic waste that accumulates during a hard workout. And finally, you need a good flexibility program in order to warm up before each workout. Often we start your workout gently and help give you time to adjust to the demands of the activity. But we don't

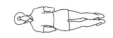

always. And even if we design the day with a warm-up, we can't know how slowly and gently you'll start that workout, or how effectively you'll warm up your muscles.

Some strength and flexibility programs are better than others. We suggest that you refer to our books *The Whartons' Strength Book* and *The Whartons' Stretch Book* for the most effective and time-efficient programs.

WHAT IF I WANT TO PARTICIPATE IN MORE THAN ONE PROGRAM?

Once you scan the workout programs, you might decide that they're so much fun, you want to participate in more than one. It's not unusual for an endurance athlete to train in two or more activities at the same time. It's called cross-training—meaning that you cross from one sport to another and back again. The method was first used to keep athletes in shape when injuries sidelined them. Instead of losing the benefits of all that good aerobic training, athletes cross to another sport of equal cardiovascular challenge. For example, an injured runner might cycle or swim to keep in shape while the injury heals sufficiently for a return to running. By the way, if this running-cycling-swimming combo sounds vaguely familiar to those of you who follow sports, you now know how triathlons got their start. Today, cross-training is used to maintain fitness levels when you can't participate in your own activity and to supplement training programs that might need a little boost. More important, cross-training adds variety and fun to a workout program.

So how do you combine activities? Obviously, many of the activities are similar, but there are specific adjustments your body has to make to each one, so each workout program has to be started at the beginning—day one. For example, if you've been running for six months and you decide to take up cycling, you have to work through and build the cycling program, starting with the first workout.

We suggest that you shuffle the workouts together like a deck of cards. Unless you're already in great shape, two full workouts on the same day are too difficult to manage and too time consuming. You can do one of two things:

1. Cut both workouts in half and do them both on the same day.

2. Do one workout on one designated training day, and the other workout the next day, but progress through each schedule only half as quickly as you would if you were concentrating on one sport.

Be very careful about overtraining. You might double your fun, but you're also doubling the load on your body. Also, if you put two different workouts back to back, you have to be mindful of the physical transitions you're asking your body to make. Take a few minutes between activities to stretch out and relax muscles that have been patterning one way before you ask them to pattern another.

Remember to do strength training on the second and fourth days of each week, and warm up before every workout with a flexibility probram!

So let's get started!

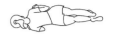

10.
The Ten Best Cardio-Fit Activities and Training Schedules

WALKING

See art, pages 1–33.

TECHNIQUE AND FORM

Most experts agree that if you're going to get one physical activity right without formal coaching, walking is it. Unless you're disabled, you've been walking since you were a toddler, and you do it very well. Likely, if you've been doing anything wrong at all, it's that you haven't been walking enough. Although proper form is important for prevention of injury and getting the most out of your workout, we think you should make it easy. Just walk. There are a few basics, however, to keep in mind. As you begin your walk, warm up a little. This means starting off slowly and gradually building to the pace at which you intend to walk. Stride evenly and smoothly. Try to begin each step by allowing your heel to strike the surface first, and then rolling forward over the ball of your foot through your toes. In other words, try to keep from slapping or flopping your feet as you walk. Keep your posture upright with your shoulders relaxed and back, and your head up. This will open up your chest so that you can breathe fully. Relax your hands. Swing your arms rhythmically as you stride: left arm with right leg and right arm with left leg—as nature intended. When you walk slowly, your arms should be down with your elbows extended and your fingertips lightly brushing your thighs. As you speed up, you'll notice your elbows naturally begin to flex and your hands come up to help you amplify, or "pump," the energy into your stride. Think of your limbs as pendulums that function in perfect opposition and synchrony to keep you moving forward and, equally important, balanced.

Be alert to your environment. Pay attention to the surface on which you are walking, so that you can make adjustments in your foot strike and avoid a stumble. Also, unless you're in a protected place (like an indoor track), keep a sharp eye out for potential dangers such as unfriendly dogs and suspicious strangers. In fact, even though music can make a workout more fun, you might want to leave your headset at home or at least leave one earpiece off so that you can stay attuned to your surroundings and listen for problems. And remember the rules of the road: on pavement, walk on the side facing traffic.

EQUIPMENT YOU'LL NEED

A watch

An identification card to put in your pocket

A bottle of water

A cell phone (possibly in a fanny pack)

WHAT TO WEAR

Dress so that you'll be comfortable and can move easily. One of the great things about walking is that it requires no special uniform. If you're walking in the evening or at night, wear light-colored clothing. Consider a reflective vest or reflectors on your shoes.

Shoes: The only clothing essential is a pair of walking shoes. Walking shoes are designed specifically to cushion the bottoms of the feet and to allow as natural a foot strike as possible in the walking gait. They are constructed differently from running, racquet, or aerobic dance shoes . . . although in a pinch, any of these shoes will do nicely. When you shop for walking shoes, take along a pair of socks like the ones you intend to wear when you walk. Also, experts suggest that you try on the shoes at the same time of day you intend to walk, because the size of your foot may vary by as much as half a size during the course of your day. When you find a pair of shoes you like, try on *both* shoes. Lace them fully, and walk around the sales floor. Make sure you can get off the carpet and onto a hard surface if you really want to get a feel for how they'll perform for you in "real life"—unless you plan to walk only on carpet when you work out. (We favor one athletic shoe store that allows us to wear the shoes outside on a clean sidewalk they maintain for this purpose.) Put the shoes through their paces—slow, fast, left turn, right turn, pivot, and about-face. Try on more than one pair and test each equally. Pay attention to raised surfaces, seams, and rough spots inside the shoe. They might seem like petty annoyances

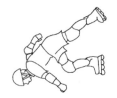

in the shoe store, but they'll turn into big problems when you start adding on the miles. Avoid being swayed by a shoe's appearance. It's what's inside and underneath that counts. In fact, we ask our clients to evaluate shoes with their eyes closed for at least a moment. In making your final decision about which shoes to buy, remember that comfort and fit are much more important than a fancy sales pitch from a clerk who may or may not be particularly knowledgeable about walking shoes and the biomechanics of walking. *You* take charge here. After all, you're going to be working out in the shoes.

Socks: Socks are optional, but most people appreciate them. They add a layer of protection between your foot and the inside of the shoe. Look for a smooth, snug fit that's free from wrinkles and inside seams. Because even the best socks are an inexpensive investment, go first-class. Purchase athletes' socks that are engineered to wick moisture, or absorb sweat away from your foot and provide you with a dryer shoe interior, which helps prevent blistering, skin irritations, and odor. Treat yourself to a clean pair of socks with every workout.

BOREDOM BUSTERS

Listen to music: Portable CD players, tape decks, and radios with lightweight headsets are popular among walkers. Just make sure that your choice of music is compatible with your planned workout. You know what we mean. Nothing trashes a good pace faster than an operatic funeral dirge. If you're walking in the company of other people who are trying to pace their own workouts, be sure you're using a headset that affords you complete privacy. In other words, do everything possible to keep from imposing (or inflicting) your choice of music—and its accompanying rhythms—on other walkers who may not share your fondness for polkas. Again, when using a headset, leave one ear totally free so that you can hear what's going on around you and stay alert to your environment. If you are walking beside a roadway, leave free the ear that is closest to traffic. Digital stereo is great, but it's dangerous in a workout.

Listen to books on tape: Raid your local library for books on tape, and improve your mind while you work out. We've known many a walker who worked his or her way through the classics while becoming fit. Follow all the rules of courtesy and safety when you're using a portable tape player with a headset.

Recruit a partner: Walking and talking go together. If you enjoy the company of a fellow walker, you'll notice that there is something very special about conversations that take place during a walk. Perhaps because the time allocated to walking is relaxed, uninterrupted, and without distractions, conversation just seems to flow. However, don't get so into your talk that you slow down below your minimum heart rate. Walking with a partner is a good idea—even if you never utter a word. There's safety in numbers, and you'll motivate each other to keep the appointment to walk. By the way, if you would like a companion who doesn't talk, but will gladly accommodate *any* workout pace and schedule you want, take your dog along. There is no finer workout partner for a walker.

Make deals: If you need a little extra incentive, try making deals with yourself—rewards for sticking to your program: "Keep this pace as far as that tree, and then I can back off until I get to that Buick." "Walk every day for a whole week, and I can have a new pair of shorts."

Be present: One of the skills most of us have lost in our hectic lives is the ability to just *be.* We're always reviewing things that have already happened or planning what's about to happen. Being in the moment is a particular challenge. Try this as you walk: just *be.* Quiet down. Try to think only of *now.* Notice the birds and squirrels. The temperature of the air. How your foot feels as it strikes the surface. The sound of your breathing. Try to experience a present moment.

Go on tour: If variety is the spice of life, then flavor your workout by changing your route. Go sightseeing. We've known some highly successful walkers who drive their cars to scout out new, more entertaining routes.

TAKING IT TO THE GYM

Indoor track

Treadmill

Stair stepper

INJURY ALERT

Walking is a gentle sport that has very few risks. If your shoes fit properly, you won't even have to worry about blisters. But if you do develop a blister, stop your workout right away. Infected blisters are trouble.

TIPS FROM THE EXPERTS

The fitness benefits of walking have been among the best-kept secrets in sports. But the truth is that walking is a powerful fat-burning, muscle-building, cardio-pumping, fitness-enhancing activity. Because walking is simple and basic, it's easy to forget that a walker is an athlete like all others. Don't make that mistake. Warm up before you work out. Train adequately before you progress from one level to the next. Be sure to hydrate before, during, and after your workouts. Be conscious of using good form. Take care of your shoes and socks. And treat small injuries and irritations immediately, before they become big ones.

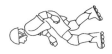

COMING TO TERMS WITH THE TERMS WE USE IN YOUR SCHEDULE

Stroll: This is a leisurely, conversational pace. You should be in the minimum range of your target heart rate. We use the stroll for helping you adjust to the gait. We want you to concentrate on perfect form and get used to your shoes.

Walk: This is a quickened pace, but still conversational. You should be in the middle range of your target heart rate.

Stride out: This is race pace. You'll be exerting effort. You should be in the higher ranges of your target heart rate.

Surfaces: If we specify the topography (such as rolling hills or flat surfaces), do your best to follow our suggestions. If working out on specific surfaces isn't possible, any surface will do. If we haven't specified a surface, choose one you like.

DAY	1	Strength Work 2	3	Strength Work 4	5	Strength Work 6	7
WEEK 1 EASY	Make sure your shoes and clothing are in order.	Stroll 15 min.	Rest.	Stroll 15 min.	Rest.	Stroll 10 min.	Stroll 15 min.
2 MODERATE	Rest.	Stroll 15 min.	Rest.	Stroll 20 min.	Rest.	Stroll 15 min.	Stroll 20 min.
3 EASY							
4 HARD							
5 EASY							
6 HARD							

WALKING BEGINNER   *1. Awakening the Body*

WALKING BEGINNER

DAY	1	2 (Strength Work)	3	4 (Strength Work)	5	6 (Strength Work)	7
WEEK 1 EASY	Rest.	Stroll 20 min.	Stroll 5 min. Stroll/Walk 20 min. (alternate strolling and walking in 5-min. intervals). Stroll 5 min.	Stroll 20 min.	Rest.	Stroll 20 min.	Stroll 5 min. Stroll/Walk 10 min. (alternate strolling and walking in 1-min. intervals). Stroll 5 min.
2 MODERATE	Rest.	Stroll 10 min. Walk 20 min. Stroll 10 min.	Stroll 20 min.	Rest.	Stroll 5 min. Stroll/Walk 10 min. (alternate strolling and walking in 1-min. intervals). Stroll 5 min.	Rest.	Stroll 10 min. Walk 5 min. Stroll 10 min.
3 EASY	Rest.	Stroll 25 min.	Rest.	Walk 25 min.	Rest.	Walk 20 min.	Stroll 5 min. Walk 5 min. Stroll 5 min. Walk 5 min. Stroll 5 min.
4 HARD	Rest.	Stroll 5 min. Walk 5 min. Stroll 5 min. Walk 5 min. Stroll 5 min.	Walk 25 min. Stroll 5 min.	Stroll 5 min. Walk 5 min. Stroll 5 min.	Rest.	Stroll 20 min.	Hill stroll: Uphill for 15 min. Downhill for 15 min.
5 EASY	Rest.	Stroll 5 min. Walk 10 min. Stroll 5 min. Walk 5 min. Stroll 5 min.	Rest.	Rest.	Stroll 5 min. Stroll/Walk 10 min. (alternate strolling and walking in 1-min. intervals). Stroll 10 min.	Rest.	Stroll 5 min. Walk 5 min. Stroll 10 min. Walk 5 min. Stroll 5 min.
6 HARD	Rest.	Hill walk: Uphill for 15 min. Downhill for 15 min.	Stroll 10 min. Walk 15 min. Stroll 10 min.	Stroll 10 min. Walk 5 min. Stroll 10 min.	Rest.	Walk 20 min.	Stroll 5 min. Walk 10 min. Stroll 10 min.

WALKING BEGINNER 2. Laying the Foundation

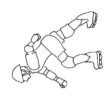

WALKING BEGINNER 3. Building Endurance

DAY	1	2 (Strength Work)	3	4 (Strength Work)	5	6 (Strength Work)	7
WEEK 1 EASY	Rest.	Rolling hill work: Stroll 5 min. Walk 5 min. Stroll 5 min. Walk 5 min. Stroll 5 min.	Stroll 5 min. Walk 10 min. Stroll 5 min.	Rest.	Rolling hill work: Stroll 5 min. Walk 10 min. Stroll 5 min. Walk 5 min. Stroll 5 min.	Rest.	Stroll 5 min. Walk 20 min. Stroll 5 min.
2 MODERATE	Rest.	Rolling hill work: Stroll 5 min. Walk 10 min. Stroll 5 min. Walk 5 min. Stroll 5 min.	Walk 5 min. Stride out 10 min. Walk 5 min.	Stroll 10 min. Stride out 10 min. Stroll 10 min.	Rest.	Stroll 5 min. Walk 15 min. Stroll 10 min.	Stroll 5 min. Walk 20 min. Stroll 5 min.
3 EASY	Rest.	Rolling hill work: Stroll 5 min. Walk 10 min. Stroll 5 min. Walk 10 min. Stroll 5 min.	Walk 5 min. Stride out 15 min. Walk 5 min.	Rest.	Rolling hill work: Stroll 15 min. Walk 15 min. Stroll 10 min.	Rest.	Walk 15 min. Stride out 20 min. Walk 5 min.
4 HARD	Rest.	Rolling hill work: Stroll 5 min. Walk 10 min. Stride out 20 min. Stroll 5 min.	Walk 5 min. Stride out 15 min. Walk 5 min.	Rolling hill work: Stroll 5 min. Walk 5 min. Stroll 5 min. Walk 10 min. Stroll 5 min.	Rolling hill work: Stroll 5 min. Walk 10 min. Stroll 5 min. Walk 5 min. Stroll 5 min.	Stroll 5 min. Walk 20 min. Stroll 5 min. Walk 5 min. Stroll 5 min.	Walk 15 min. Stride out 25 min. Walk 5 min.
5 EASY	Rest.	Rolling hill work: Stroll 5 min. Walk 15 min. Stroll 5 min. Walk 10 min. Stroll 5 min.	Walk 5 min. Stride out 20 min. Walk 5 min.	Rest.	Rolling hill work: Stroll 5 min. Walk 10 min. Stroll 5 min. Walk 5 min. Stroll 5 min.	Rest.	Walk 25 min.
6 HARD	Rest.	Rolling hill work: Stroll 5 min. Walk 10 min. Stroll 5 min. Walk 15 min. Stroll 5 min.	Walk 15 min. Stride out 25 min. Walk 5 min.	Stroll 5 min. Walk 5 min. Stroll 5 min. Walk 5 min. Stroll 5 min.	Rest.	Walk 5 min. Stride out 10 min. Walk 5 min.	Walk 30 min.

WALKING BEGINNER 4. Achieving Mastery

DAY	1	Strength Work 2	3	Strength Work 4	5	Strength Work 6	7
WEEK 1 EASY	Rest.	Rolling hill work: Walk 5 min. Stride out 25 min. Walk 5 min.	On flat surface: Walk 5 min. Stride out 15 min. Walk 5 min. Stride out 10 min. Walk 5 min.	Rest.	Rolling hill work: Walk 5 min. Stride out 5 min. Walk 5 min. Repeat entire pattern.	On flat surface: Walk 5 min. Stride out 20 min. Walk 5 min.	On flat surface: Walk 5 min. Stride out 20 min. Walk 5 min.
2 MODERATE	Rest.	Rolling hill work: Walk 5 min. Stride out 25 min. Walk 5 min.	On flat surface: Walk 5 min. Stride out 10 min. Walk 5 min. Stride out 10 min. Walk 5 min.	Rolling hill work: Walk 5 min. Stride out 15 min. Walk 5 min. Stride out 10 min. Walk 5 min.	Rest.	Rolling hill work: Walk 10 min. Stride out 15 min. Walk 5 min.	On flat surface: Walk 20 min. Stride out 10 min. Walk 10 min.
3 EASY							
4 HARD							
5 EASY							
6 HARD							

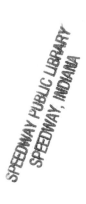

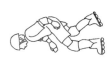

WALKING INTERMEDIATE 5. Awakening the Body

DAY	1	Strength Work 2	3	4	5	Strength Work 6	7
WEEK 1 EASY	Rest.	On flat surface: Walk 5 min. Stride out 25 min. Walk 5 min.	Walk 5 min. Stride out 10 min. Walk 5 min. Stride out 10 min. Walk 5 min.	Rolling hill work: Walk 5 min. Stride out 15 min. Walk 5 min. Stride out 10 min. Walk 5 min.	Rest.	Rolling hill work: Walk 10 min. Stride out 15 min. Walk 5 min.	Rolling hill work: Walk 20 min. Stride out 10 min. Walk 10 min.
2 MODERATE	Rest.	Rolling hill work: Walk 10 min. Stride out 25 min. Walk 10 min.	Walk 5 min. Stride out 15 min. Walk 5 min. Stride out 15 min. Walk 5 min.	Rolling hill work: Walk 10 min. For 30 min., alternate 1 min. walking with 1 min. striding. Walk 5 min.	Rest.	Rolling hill work: Walk 10 min. Stride out 20 min. Walk 5 min.	Hill work: Stride out uphill 20 min. Stride out downhill 15 min.
3 EASY							
4 HARD							
5 EASY							
6 HARD							

WALKING INTERMEDIATE *6. Laying the Foundation*

DAY	1	Strength Work 2	3	4	5	Strength Work 6	7
WEEK 1 EASY	Rest.	Rolling hill work: Walk 30 min.	Walk 5 min. Stride out 15 min. Walk 5 min. Stride out 15 min. Walk 5 min.	Rolling hill work: Stroll 10 min. For 25 min., alternate 1 min. walking with 1 min. striding. Walk 5 min.	Rest.	Rolling hill work: Walk 10 min. Stride out 20 min. Walk 5 min.	Hill work: Alternate walking and striding: Uphill 20 min. Downhill 15 min.
2 MODERATE	Rest.	Rolling hill work: Walk 20 min. Stride out 10 min. Walk 5 min.	Walk 5 min. Stride out 20 min. Walk 5 min. Stride out 10 min. Walk 5 min.	Rolling hill work: Walk 5 min. For 35 min., alternate 5 min. walking with 5 min. striding. Walk 5 min.	Rest.	Rolling hill work: Walk 5 min. Stride out 25 min. Walk 5 min.	Hill work: Alternate walking and striding: Uphill 25 min. Downhill 20 min.
3 EASY	Rest.	Rolling hill work: Walk 15 min. Stride out 10 min. Walk 5 min.	On flat surface: Walk 5 min. Stride out 15 min. Walk 5 min. Stride out 10 min. Walk 5 min.	Rolling hill work: Walk 5 min. For 35 min., alternate 5 min. walking with 5 min. striding. Walk 5 min.	Rest.	Rolling hill work: Walk 35 min.	Hill work: Alternate walking and striding: Uphill 25 min. Downhill 20 min.
4 HARD	Rest.	Rolling hill work: Walk 30 min. Stride out 15 min. Walk 5 min.	Walk 5 min. Stride out 20 min. Walk 5 min. Stride out 10 min. Walk 5 min.	Rolling hill work: Walk 5 min. For 35 min., alternate 1 min. walking with 1 min. striding. Walk 5 min.	Rest.	Rolling hill work: Stride out 25 min. Walk 5 min.	Hill work: Alternate walking and striding: Uphill 25 min. Downhill 20 min.
5 EASY	Rest.	Rolling hill work: Walk 10 min. Stride out 10 min. Walk 5 min.	Walk 10 min. Stride out 10 min. Walk 5 min. Stride out 5 min. Walk 5 min.	Rolling hill work: Walk 5 min. For 35 min., alternate 5 min. walking with 5 min. striding. Walk 5 min.	Rest.	Rolling hill work: Walk 5 min. Stride out 25 min. Walk 5 min.	Hill work: Alternate walking and striding: Uphill 25 min. Downhill 20 min.
6 HARD	Rest.	Rolling hill work: Walk 10 min. Stride out 20 min. Walk 5 min.	Walk 10 min. Stride out 20 min. Walk 5 min. Stride out 5 min. Walk 5 min.	Rolling hill work: Walk 5 min. For 35 min., alternate 5 min. walking with 5 min. striding. Walk 5 min.	Rest.	Rolling hill work: Stride out 30 min. Walk 5 min.	Rolling hill work: Walk 10 min. Stride out 20 min. Walk 5 min. Stride out 5 min. Walk 5 min.

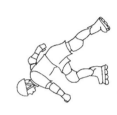

DAY	1	Strength Work 2	Strength Work 3	Strength Work 4	5	Strength Work 6	7
WEEK 1 EASY	Rest.	Rolling hill work: Stride out 15 min. Walk 5 min.	Rolling hill work: Walk 10 min. Stride out 10 min. Walk 5 min.	Rolling hill work: Stride out 5 min. Walk 2 min. Stride out 5 min. Walk 5 min.	Rest.	Walk 20 min. Stride out 5 min. Walk 5 min.	Rolling hill work: Walk 30 min.
2 MODERATE	Rest.	Rolling hill work: Stride out 15 min. Walk 5 min.	Rolling hill work: Walk 10 min. Stride out 10 min. Walk 5 min.	Rolling hill work: Stride out 5 min. Walk 2 min. Stride out 10 min. Walk 5 min.	Rest.	Walk 15 min. Stride out 10 min. Walk 5 min.	Rolling hill work: Stride out 30 min.
3 EASY	Rest.	Rolling hill work: Stride out 15 min. Walk 5 min.	Rolling hill work: Walk 15 min. Stride out 10 min. Walk 5 min.	Rolling hill work: Stride out 5 min. Walk 2 min. Stride out 10 min. Walk 5 min.	Rest.	Walk 20 min. Stride out 5 min. Walk 5 min.	Rolling hill work: Stride out 30 min.
4 HARD	Rest.	Rolling hill work: Stride out 20 min. Walk 5 min.	Rolling hill work: Walk 15 min. Stride out 10 min. Walk 5 min.	Rolling hill work: Stride out 5 min. Walk 2 min. Stride out 7 min. Walk 5 min.	Rest.	Walk 20 min. Stride out 10 min. Walk 5 min.	Rolling hill work: Stride out 30 min.
5 EASY	Rest.	Rolling hill work: Stride out 20 min. Walk 5 min.	Rolling hill work: Walk 15 min. Stride out 10 min. Walk 5 min.	Rolling hill work: Stride out 5 min. Walk 2 min. Stride out 7 min. Walk 5 min.	Rest.	Walk 20 min. Stride out 10 min. Walk 5 min.	Rolling hill work: Stride out 35 min.
6 HARD	Rest.	Rolling hill work: Stride out 25 min. Walk 5 min.	Rest.	Rolling hill work: Stride out 10 min. Walk 2 min. Stride out 10 min. Walk 5 min.	Rest.	Walk 30 min.	Rolling hill work: Stride out 35 min.

WALKING INTERMEDIATE *7. Building Endurance*

WALKING INTERMEDIATE 8. Achieving Mastery

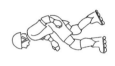

DAY	1	Strength Work 2	3	Strength Work 4	5	Strength Work 6	7
WEEK 1 EASY	Rest.	Rolling hill work: Stride out 35 min.	Rolling hill work: Walk 5 min. Stride out 5 min. Stride out 7 min. Walk 5 min.	Rolling hill work: Walk 10 min. Stride out 10 min. Walk 10 min.	Rest.	Walk 15 min. Stride out 10 min. Walk 2 min.	Rolling hill work: Stride out 35 min. Walk 5 min.
2 MODERATE	Rest.	Rolling hill work: Stride out 35 min.	Rolling hill work: Walk 5 min. Stride out 10 min. Walk 5 min. Stride out 7 min. Walk 5 min.	Rolling hill work: Stride out 25 min. Walk 5 min.	Rest.	Walk 20 min. Stride out 10 min. Walk 2 min.	Rolling hill work: Stride out 35 min. Walk 5 min.
3 EASY	Rest.	Rolling hill work: Stride out 35 min.	Rest.	Rolling hill work: Stride out 20 min. Walk 5 min.	Rest.	Walk 15 min. Stride out 10 min. Walk 2 min.	Rolling hill work: Stride out 35 min. Walk 5 min.
4 HARD	Rest.	Rolling hill work: Stride out 35 min.	Rolling hill work: Stride out 20 min. Walk 5 min.	Rolling hill work: Stride out 25 min. Walk 5 min.	Rest.	Walk 10 min. Stride out 20 min. Walk 2 min.	Rolling hill work: Stride out 35 min. Walk 5 min.
5 EASY							
6 HARD							

DAY	1	Strength Work 2	3	Strength Work 4	5	Strength Work 6	7
WEEK 1 EASY	Rest.	Rolling hill work: Stride out 25 min. Walk 5 min.	Walk 10 min. Stride out 20 min. Walk 5 min.	Walk 5 min. Stride out 15 min. Walk 10 min.	Rest.	Walk 20 min. Stride out 20 min. Walk 5 min.	Rolling hill work: Stride out 45 min. Walk 5 min.
2 MODERATE	Rest.	Rolling hill work: Stride out 30 min. Walk 5 min.	Rest.	Rolling hill work: Stride out 25 min. Walk 5 min.	Rest.	Walk 40 min.	Rolling hill work: Stride out 45 min. Walk 5 min.
3 EASY							
4 HARD							
5 EASY							
6 HARD							

WALKING ADVANCED *9. Awakening the Body*

DAY	1	Strength Work 2	3	Strength Work 4	5	Strength Work 6	7
WEEK 1 EASY	Rest.	Rolling hill work: Stride out 35 min. Walk 5 min.	Rolling hill work: Walk 5 min. Stride out 30 min. Walk 5 min.	Stride out 15 min. Pick up your pace 10 min. Stride out 5 min.	Rest.	Walk 20 min. Stride out 20 min.	Rolling hill work: Stride out 40 min. Walk 5 min.
2 MODERATE	Rest.	Rolling hill work: Stride out 35 min. Walk 5 min.	Rolling hill work: Walk 5 min. Stride out 40 min. Walk 5 min.	Stride out 20 min. Pick up your pace 10 min. Stride out 5 min.	Rest.	Stride out 40 min.	Rolling hill work: Stride out 40 min. Walk 5 min.
3 EASY	Rest.	Rolling hill work: Stride out 35 min. Walk 5 min.	Rest.	Stride out 20 min. Pick up your pace 10 min. Stride out 5 min.	Rest.	Walk 20 min. Stride out 30 min.	Rolling hill work: Stride out 40 min. Walk 5 min.
4 HARD	Rest.	Rolling hill work: Stride out 35 min. Walk 5 min.	Rolling hill work: Walk 5 min. Stride out 40 min. Walk 5 min.	Stride out 25 min. Pick up your pace 15 min. Stride out 5 min.	Rest.	Walk 10 min. Stride out 20 min.	Rolling hill work: Stride out 40 min. Walk 5 min.
5 EASY	Rest.	Rolling hill work: Stride out 35 min. Walk 5 min.	Game Day.	Walk 20 min. Stride out 20 min.	Rest.	Walk 20 min. Stride out 20 min.	Rolling hill work: Stride out 40 min. Walk 5 min.
6 HARD	Rest.	Rolling hill work: Stride out 35 min. Walk 5 min.	Game Day.	Walk 15 min. Stride out 30 min.	Rest.	Walk 20 min. Stride out 20 min.	Rolling hill work: Stride out 40 min. Walk 5 min.

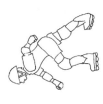

WALKING ADVANCED *10. Laying the Foundation*

WALKING ADVANCED   *11. Building Endurance*

DAY / WEEK	1	Strength Work 2	3	Strength Work 4	5	Strength Work 6	7
1 EASY	Rest.	Stride out 35 min. Keep a steady pace.	Game Day.	Walk 10 min. Stride out 30 min. Walk 5 min.	Rest.	Walk 20 min. Stride out 20 min.	Stride out 45 min. Keep a steady pace.
2 MODERATE	Rest.	Stride out 40 min. Keep a steady pace.	Game Day.	Walk 5 min. Stride out 40 min. Walk 5 min.	Rest.	Walk 20 min. Stride out 20 min.	Stride out 45 min. Keep a steady pace.
3 EASY	Rest.	Stride out 35 min. Keep a steady pace.	Game Day.	Stride out 45 min. Walk 5 min.	Rest.	Walk 20 min. Stride out 20 min.	Stride out 45 min. Keep a steady pace.
4 HARD	Rest.	Stride out 45 min. Keep a steady pace.	Game Day.	Stride out 45 min. Walk 5 min.	Rest.	Walk 20 min. Stride out 20 min.	Stride out 50 min. Keep a steady pace.
5 EASY	Rest.	Walk 5 min. Stride out 15 min. Walk 5 min. Stride out 15 min. Walk 5 min.	Stride out 40 min. Keep a steady pace.	Game Day.	Rest.	Stride out 30 min. Keep a steady pace.	Stride out 45 min. Keep a steady pace.
6 HARD	Rest.	Walk 5 min. Stride out 20 min. Walk 5 min. Stride out 20 min. Walk 5 min.	Stride out 45 min. Keep a steady pace.	Game Day.	Rest.	Stride out 30 min. Keep a steady pace.	Stride out 50 min. Keep a steady pace.

DAY	1	Strength Work 2	3	Strength Work 4	5	Strength Work 6	7
WEEK 1 EASY	Rest.	Walk 5 min. Stride out 20 min. Walk 5 min. Stride out 10 min. Walk 5 min.	Stride out 40 min.	Game Day.	Rest.	Stride out 30 min.	Stride out 45 min. Pick up the pace.
2 MODERATE	Rest.	Walk 5 min. Stride out 25 min. Walk 5 min. Stride out 5 min. Walk 5 min.	Stride out 50 min.	Game Day.	Rest.	Stride out 30 min.	Stride out 55 min. Pick up the pace.
3 EASY	Rest.	Walk 5 min. Stride out 35 min. Walk 10 min.	Stride out 30 min.	Game Day.	Rest.	Stride out 30 min.	Stride out 55 min. Pick up the pace.
4 HARD	Rest.	Stride out 35 min.	Stride out 40 min.	Stride out 30 min.	Rest.	Stride out 30 min.	Stride out 60 min. Pick up the pace.
5 EASY							
6 HARD							

WALKING ADVANCED   12. *Achieving Mastery*

RACEWALKING

See art, pages 35–65.

TECHNIQUE AND FORM

The first time people see a racewalker, their first impressions are that it looks prissy, it's just fast walking, and it can't be all that tough. These impressions might last until a Wharton assures you otherwise, or you try racewalking yourself. Either way, a second look gives you respect for the sport.

Racewalking is distinguished from running in that there is no airborne phase in the gait: one foot is always on the ground. You can't lift your rear foot and bring it into a step until your front foot is firmly in contact with the surface. Racewalking is distinguished from walking in that the whole time your foot is on the ground, the knee of that leg has to be straight. The strain on that leg is enormous as you move your body forward over the foot on the ground with as long a stride as possible. While you're moving over the grounded foot, your rear foot is straining to stay on the ground until the stride is completed. Only then can your rear foot break contact. This phase requires extreme flexibility of your foot and ankle, and places great stress on the back of your leg. Like a sprinter, you clench your fists and pump with your arms to achieve momentum by amplifying the action of your lower body. Unlike a sprinter, however, you are restricted to a completely upright posture. No leaning forward is allowed. It's one of the real challenges of the sport, because it's in direct contrast to the physics of walking as we understand it.

Walking has been described as controlled falling. Essentially, you lean forward until you are about to fall and, at the last possible moment, you stick out one foot to catch yourself: this is a step. Balance on that one foot and lean forward until you start to fall and then catch yourself with the other foot, and so on. The farther forward you lean and the more aggressive your catch, the faster you walk until you are going so fast that you anticipate the fall and prepare for it by picking up your back foot before you've passed your torso over the front foot. When both feet are off the ground at the same time, you've entered the running (airborne) phase. So how do you achieve speed when you can neither lean forward nor get airborne? The hip swing. By using that turbocharge at the hip, you get that slight forward thrust for momentum. It literally pops your back leg forward.

EQUIPMENT YOU'LL NEED

A watch

A bottle of water

An identification card to put into your pocket

Cell phone (possibly in a fanny pack)

WHAT TO WEAR

In warm weather, wear shorts and a T-shirt or singlet. Make sure they're made of lightweight material designed to keep you cool and wick sweat away from your body. Additionally, they should be loose enough to be comfortable but snug enough to avoid rubbing and blistering. By the way, if you have trouble with clothing that rubs, wear it inside out so the seams are away from your skin. With T-shirts, you might try chopping off the sleeves and neckline, eliminating the offending seams.

In cool weather, you can wear running tights under your shorts, or eliminate the shorts completely and go with the tights alone. If it's really cold outside, layering is always best. In extreme weather, you can add long pants that are specifically designed for runners. They are made to insulate you from the cold and wick sweat away. They have zippers at the bottom of each leg so you can put them on and get them off easily over your shoes. They're loose enough so you can move, but fitted and soft to keep from rubbing. Keep the T-shirt or singlet, but cover it with a long-sleeved T-shirt, sweatshirt, or weatherproof jacket that can be removed and tied around your waist if you get too hot. Wear a snugly fitting knit hat that you can pull down over your ears. Wear cotton gloves, or gloves made from silk or polypropylene that will wick sweat away from your skin. If you don't have gloves, wear an extra pair of tube socks over your hands.

Shoes: You need a pair of running shoes with good support and motion control in the heel (to keep your ankle stable). Remember that your heel will strike the ground first and the hardest. When you shop for shoes, take along a pair of socks like the ones you intend to wear when you racewalk. Also, experts suggest that you try on the shoes at the same time of day you intend to work out, because the size of your foot may vary by as much as half a size during the course of your day. When you find a pair of shoes you like, try on *both* shoes. Lace them fully, and walk around the sales floor. Make sure you can get off the carpet and onto a hard surface if you really want to get a feel for how they'll perform for you in "real life"—unless you plan to racewalk only on carpet when you train. (We favor one athletic shoe store that allows us to wear the shoes outside on a clean sidewalk they maintain for this purpose.) Put the shoes through their paces—slow, fast, left turn, right turn, pivot, and about-face. Try on more than one pair and test each equally. Pay attention to raised surfaces, seams, and rough spots inside the shoe. They might seem like petty annoyances in the shoe store, but they'll turn into big problems when you start adding on the miles. Avoid being swayed by a shoe's appearance. It's what's inside and underneath that counts. In fact, we ask our clients to evaluate shoes with their eyes closed for at least a moment. In making your final decision about which shoes to buy, remember that comfort and fit are much more important than a fancy sales pitch from a clerk who may or may not be particularly knowledgeable about shoes and the biomechanics of racewalking. *You* take charge here. After all, you're going to be working out in the shoes.

Socks: Socks are optional, but most people enjoy wearing them. They add a layer of protection between your foot and the inside of the shoe. Look for a smooth, snug fit that's free from wrinkles and inside seams. Because even the best socks are an inexpensive investment, go first-class. Purchase athletes' socks that are engineered to wick moisture, or absorb sweat, away from your foot and provide you with a dryer shoe interior, which will help prevent blistering, skin irritations, and odor. Treat yourself to a clean pair of socks with every workout.

Undergarments: Although racewalking is a fairly fluid activity, it still causes a wiggle here and a jiggle there. Both men and women should wear undergarments that support and protect delicate tissues.

BOREDOM BUSTERS

Listen to music: Portable CD and tape players and radios with lightweight headsets are popular among racewalkers. Just make sure that your choice of music is compatible with your planned workout. You know what we mean. Nothing trashes a good pace faster than an operatic funeral dirge. If you're walking in the company of other people who are trying to pace their own workouts, be sure you're using a headset that affords you complete privacy. In other words, do everything possible to keep from imposing (or inflicting) your choice of music—and its accompanying rhythms—on other racewalkers. When using a headset, leave one ear totally free so that you can hear what's going on around you and stay alert to your environment. If you're racewalking beside a roadway, leave free the ear that is closest to traffic. Digital stereo is great, but it's dangerous in a workout.

Listen to books on tape: Raid your local library for books on tape, and improve your mind while you work out. We've known many a racewalker who worked his or her way through the classics while becoming fit. Follow all the rules of courtesy and safety when you're using a portable tape player with a headset.

Recruit a partner: For athletes who train outside on streets or on tracks, there's safety in numbers. There's also motivation. You and a friend can work together to keep your training schedules on track. Better yet, join a club where you can work out with other racewalkers and coaches who share your passion and will help you improve.

Sign up for a race: Nothing motivates a racewalker like an upcoming competition. Targeting a specific goal on a specific date puts focus and excitement into even the most anemic program. Don't be discouraged if you can't find events for racewalking. Yours is a hybrid sport. Any event that is designed for runners or walkers is also designed for you, even a marathon.

Play utility poles: This is a favorite game among runners who use it to introduce speed work, or "tempo," into their training. It adapts spectacularly to racewalking. Utility poles are good gauges of precise distance because they are evenly placed in the ground beside the road. Pick up your pace from one pole to the next, then back off until you reach the third pole. Pick up your pace again, and so on and so on. As you develop stamina, try increasing the numbers of poles between which you pick up your pace, such as picking up the pace for three poles, and backing off one pole.

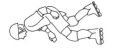

Urban touring: This is a game developed by Phil for himself and his runner-friends who live and train in New York City. It adapts very well to racewalking. The only requirements are city sidewalks and traffic lights. The point of the game is to travel as far as you can without stopping. Racewalk straight down the sidewalk. When you inevitably encounter a stoplight that could impede you from continuing your route, don't stop. Immediately change direction. Go either right or left, and continue straight along that route until you encounter another stoplight. Don't stop. Follow the "Walk" signal. Look *both* ways first. Change direction. You'll never be sure where you'll be led to travel, and you'll have to make some quick decisions that will take you on an undetermined, random journey. (Phil notes that the game becomes really challenging when you decide it's time to get home.)

TAKING IT TO THE GYM

Indoor track

Treadmill

INJURY ALERT

Injuries in racewalking are generally of the lower extremities: muscles along the tibia tend to strain if the ankles and feet are inflexible, and the athlete has difficulty in keeping the rear foot on the ground. (You'll soon see why we discourage racewalking as an alternative for a runner with a tibial stress fracture.) The extreme trunk rotation places an athlete at risk for strains in the lower back and abdominal muscle groups. And the straight-leg technique, as we said, places great strain on the back of the leg—specifically the Achilles tendon, the gastrocs, and the hamstring attachment at the back of your knee. Injury prevention is a function of strength and flexibility training combined with good technique. Supplemental training should include upper body work and flexibility.

TIPS FROM THE EXPERTS

Please remember to hydrate. Racewalking is a strenuous sport in both training and competition. Even slight dehydration lowers the circulating volume of blood and causes your core temperature to rise. The more dehydrated the athlete becomes, the more dangerous the situation gets. Symptoms of progressive dehydration include fatigue, lack of coordination, muscle pain and cramping, headache, light-headedness, confusion, disorientation, and fainting. Under extreme circumstances, death can occur. If you feel thirsty, you're already on your way to trouble. Drink early—before thirst sets in—and often. Experts say that water is perfect for short events, but a commercial sport fluid-replacement drink is preferable for events of more than ninety minutes in duration. With either choice, *cold* is best. We want you to play it cool. Drink.

COMING TO TERMS WITH THE TERMS WE USE IN YOUR SCHEDULE

Stroll: This is a leisurely, conversational pace. You should be in the minimum range of your target heart rate. We use the stroll for helping you adjust to the gait. We want you to concentrate on perfect form and get used to your shoes.

Walk: This is a quickened pace, but still conversational. You should be in the middle range of your target heart rate.

Stride out: This is race pace. You'll be exerting effort. You should be in the higher ranges of your target heart rate.

Surfaces: If we specify the topography (such as rolling hills or flat surfaces), do your best to follow our suggestions. If working out on specific surfaces isn't possible, any surface will do. If we haven't specified a surface, choose one you like.

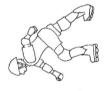

RACEWALKING BEGINNER   *1. Awakening the Body*

DAY	1	2	3	4	5	6	7
WEEK		Strength Work		Strength Work		Strength Work	
1 EASY	Make sure your shoes and clothing are in order.	Stroll 15 min.	Rest.	Stroll 15 min.	Rest.	Stroll 10 min.	Stroll 15 min.
2 MODERATE	Rest.	Stroll 15 min.	Rest.	Stroll 20 min.	Rest.	Stroll 15 min.	Stroll 20 min.
3 EASY							
4 HARD							
5 EASY							
6 HARD							

DAY	1	Strength Work 2	3	Strength Work 4	5	Strength Work 6	7
WEEK 1 EASY	Rest.	Stroll 20 min.	Stroll 5 min. Stroll/Walk 20 min. (alternate strolling and Walking in 5-min. intervals). Stroll 5 min.	Stroll 20 min.	Rest.	Stroll 20 min.	Stroll 5 min. Stroll/Walk 10 min. (alternate strolling and walking in 1-min. intervals). Stroll 5 min.
2 MODERATE	Rest.	Stroll 10 min. Walk 20 min. Stroll 10 min.	Stroll 20 min.	Rest.	Stroll 5 min. Stroll/Walk 10 min. (alternate strolling and walking in 1-min. intervals). Stroll 5 min.	Rest.	Stroll 10 min. Walk 5 min. Stroll 10 min.
3 EASY	Rest.	Stroll 25 min.	Rest.	Walk 25 min.	Rest.	Walk 20 min.	Stroll 5 min. Walk 5 min. Stroll 5 min. Stroll 5 min.
4 HARD	Rest.	Stroll 5 min. Walk 5 min. Stroll 5 min. Walk 5 min. Stroll 5 min.	Walk 25 min. Stroll 5 min.	Stroll 5 min. Walk 5 min. Stroll 5 min.	Rest.	Stroll 20 min.	Hill stroll: Uphill for 15 min. Downhill for 15 min.
5 EASY	Rest.	Stroll 5 min. Walk 10 min. Stroll 5 min. Walk 5 min. Stroll 5 min.	Rest.	Rest.	Stroll 5 min. Stroll/Walk 10 min. (alternate strolling and walking in 1-min. intervals). Stroll 10 min.	Rest.	Stroll 5 min. Walk 10 min. Stroll 10 min.
6 HARD	Rest.	Hill walk: Uphill for 15 min. Downhill for 15 min.	Stroll 10 min. Walk 15 min. Stroll 10 min.	Stroll 10 min. Walk 5 min. Stroll 10 min.	Rest.	Walk 20 min.	Stroll 5 min. Walk 10 min. Stroll 10 min.

RACEWALKING BEGINNER 2. Laying the Foundation

RACEWALKING BEGINNER 3. *Building Endurance*

DAY / WEEK	1	Strength Work 2	3	Strength Work 4	5	Strength Work 6	7
1 EASY	Rest.	Rolling hill work: Stroll 5 min. Walk 5 min. Stroll 5 min. Walk 5 min. Stroll 5 min.	Stroll 5 min. Walk 10 min. Stroll 5 min.	Rest.	Rolling hill work: Stroll 5 min. Walk 10 min. Stroll 5 min. Walk 5 min. Stroll 5 min.	Rest.	Stroll 5 min. Walk 20 min. Stroll 5 min.
2 MODERATE	Rest.	Rolling hill work: Stroll 5 min. Walk 10 min. Stroll 5 min. Walk 5 min. Stroll 5 min.	Walk 5 min. Stride out 10 min. Walk 5 min.	Stroll 10 min. Stride out 10 min. Stroll 10 min.	Rest.	Stroll 5 min. Walk 15 min. Stroll 10 min.	Stroll 5 min. Walk 20 min. Stroll 5 min.
3 EASY	Rest.	Rolling hill work: Stroll 5 min. Walk 10 min. Stroll 5 min. Walk 10 min. Stroll 5 min.	Walk 5 min. Stride out 15 min. Walk 5 min.	Rest.	Rolling hill work: Stroll 15 min. Walk 15 min. Stroll 10 min.	Rest.	Walk 15 min. Stride out 20 min. Walk 5 min.
4 HARD	Rest.	Rolling hill work: Stroll 5 min. Stride out 20 min. Stroll 5 min.	Walk 5 min. Stride out 15 min. Walk 5 min.	Rolling hill work: Stroll 5 min. Walk 5 min. Stroll 5 min. Walk 10 min. Stroll 5 min.	Rest.	Stroll 5 min. Walk 20 min. Stroll 5 min. Walk 5 min.	Walk 15 min. Stride out 25 min. Walk 5 min.
5 EASY	Rest.	Rolling hill work: Stroll 5 min. Walk 15 min. Stroll 5 min. Walk 10 min. Stroll 5 min.	Walk 5 min. Stride out 20 min. Walk 5 min.	Rest.	Rolling hill work: Stroll 5 min. Walk 10 min. Stroll 5 min. Walk 5 min. Stroll 5 min.	Rest.	Walk 25 min.
6 HARD	Rest.	Rolling hill work: Stroll 5 min. Walk 10 min. Stroll 5 min. Walk 15 min. Stroll 5 min.	Walk 15 min. Stride out 25 min. Walk 5 min.	Stroll 5 min. Walk 5 min. Stroll 5 min. Walk 5 min. Stroll 5 min.	Rest.	Walk 5 min. Stride out 10 min. Walk 5 min.	Walk 30 min.

DAY	1	2	3	4	5	6	7
		Strength Work		Strength Work		Strength Work	
WEEK							
1 EASY	Rest.	Rolling hill work: Walk 5 min. Stride out 25 min. Walk 5 min.	On flat surface: Walk 5 min. Stride out 15 min. Walk 5 min. Stride out 10 min. Walk 5 min.	Rest.	Rolling hill work: Walk 5 min. Stride out 5 min. Walk 5 min. Repeat entire pattern.	On flat surface: Walk 5 min. Stride out 20 min. Walk 5 min.	On flat surface: Walk 5 min. Stride out 20 min. Walk 5 min.
2 MODERATE	Rest.	Rolling hill work: Walk 5 min. Stride out 25 min. Walk 5 min.	On flat surface: Walk 5 min. Stride out 10 min. Walk 5 min. Stride out 10 min. Walk 5 min.	Rolling hill work: Walk 5 min. Stride out 15 min. Walk 5 min. Stride out 10 min. Walk 5 min.	Rest.	Rolling hill work: Walk 10 min. Stride out 15 min. Walk 5 min.	On flat surface: Walk 20 min. Stride out 10 min. Walk 10 min.
3 EASY							
4 HARD							
5 EASY							
6 HARD							

RACEWALKING BEGINNER *4. Achieving Mastery*

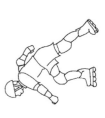

DAY	1	Strength Work 2	3	Strength Work 4	5	Strength Work 6	7
WEEK 1 EASY	Rest.	On flat surface: Walk 5 min. Stride out 25 min. Walk 5 min.	Walk 5 min. Stride out 10 min. Walk 5 min. Stride out 10 min. Walk 5 min.	Rolling hill work: Walk 5 min. Stride out 15 min. Walk 5 min. Stride out 10 min. Walk 5 min.	Rest.	Rolling hill work: Walk 10 min. Stride out 15 min. Walk 5 min.	Rolling hill work: Walk 20 min. Stride out 10 min. Walk 10 min.
2 MODERATE	Rest.	Rolling hill work: Walk 10 min. Stride out 25 min. Walk 10 min.	Walk 5 min. Stride out 15 min. Walk 5 min. Stride out 15 min. Walk 5 min.	Rolling hill work: Walk 10 min. For 30 min., alternate 1 min. walking with 1 min. striding. Walk 5 min.	Rest.	Rolling hill work: Walk 10 min. Stride out 20 min. Walk 5 min.	Hill work: Stride out uphill 20 min. Stride out downhill 15 min.
3 EASY							
4 HARD							
5 EASY							
6 HARD							

RACEWALKING INTERMEDIATE 5. Awakening the Body

DAY	1	Strength Work 2	3	Strength Work 4	5	Strength Work 6	7
WEEK 1 EASY	Rest.	Rolling hill work: Walk 30 min.	Walk 5 min. Stride out 15 min. Walk 5 min. Stride out 15 min. Walk 5 min.	Rolling hill work: Stroll 10 min. For 25 min. alternate 1 min. walking with 1 min. striding. Walk 5 min.	Rest.	Rolling hill work: Walk 10 min. Stride out 20 min. Walk 5 min.	Hill work: Alternate walking and striding: Uphill 20 min. Downhill 15 min.
2 MODERATE	Rest.	Rolling hill work: Walk 20 min. Stride out 10 min. Walk 5 min.	Walk 5 min. Stride out 20 min. Walk 5 min. Stride out 10 min. Walk 5 min.	Rolling hill work: Walk 5 min. For 35 min., alternate 5 min. walking with 5 min. striding. Walk 5 min.	Rest.	Rolling hill work: Walk 5 min. Stride out 25 min. Walk 5 min.	Hill work: Alternate walking and striding: Uphill 25 min. Downhill 20 min.
3 EASY	Rest.	Rolling hill work: Walk 15 min. Stride out 10 min. Walk 5 min.	On flat surface: Walk 5 min. Stride out 15 min. Walk 5 min. Stride out 10 min. Walk 5 min.	Rolling hill work: Walk 5 min. For 35 min., alternate 5 min. walking with 5 min. striding. Walk 5 min.	Rest.	Rolling hill work: Walk 35 min.	Hill work: Alternate walking and striding: Uphill 25 min. Downhill 20 min.
4 HARD	Rest.	Rolling hill work: Walk 30 min. Stride out 15 min. Walk 5 min.	Walk 5 min. Stride out 20 min. Walk 5 min. Stride out 10 min. Walk 5 min.	Rolling hill work: Walk 5 min. For 35 min., alternate 1 min. walking with 1 min. striding. Walk 5 min.	Rest.	Rolling hill work: Stride out 25 min. Walk 5 min.	Hill work: Alternate walking and striding: Uphill 25 min. Downhill 20 min.
5 EASY	Rest.	Rolling hill work: Walk 10 min. Stride out 10 min. Walk 5 min.	Walk 10 min. Stride out 5 min. Walk 5 min.	Rolling hill work: Walk 5 min. For 35 min., alternate 5 min. walking with 5 min. striding. Walk 5 min.	Rest.	Rolling hill work: Walk 5 min. Stride out 25 min. Walk 5 min.	Hill work: Alternate walking and striding: Uphill 25 min. Downhill 20 min.
6 HARD	Rest.	Rolling hill work: Walk 10 min. Stride out 20 min. Walk 5 min.	Walk 10 min. Stride out 5 min. Walk 5 min.	Rolling hill work: Walk 5 min. For 35 min., alternate 5 min. walking with 5 min. striding. Walk 5 min.	Rest.	Rolling hill work: Stride out 30 min. Walk 5 min.	Hill work: Walk 10 min. Stride out 20 min. Walk 5 min. Stride out 5 min. Walk 5 min.

RACEWALKING INTERMEDIATE 6. *Laying the Foundation*

RACEWALKING INTERMEDIATE 7. *Building Endurance*

DAY	1	2 Strength Work	3	4 Strength Work	5	6 Strength Work	7 Strength Work
WEEK 1 EASY	Rest.	Rolling hill work: Stride out 15 min. Walk 5 min.	Rolling hill work: Walk 10 min. Stride out 10 min. Walk 5 min.	Rolling hill work: Stride out 5 min. Walk 2 min. Stride out 5 min. Walk 5 min.	Rest.	Walk 20 min. Stride out 5 min. Walk 5 min.	Rolling hill work: Walk 30 min.
2 MODERATE	Rest.	Rolling hill work: Stride out 15 min. Walk 5 min.	Rolling hill work: Walk 10 min. Stride out 10 min. Walk 5 min.	Rolling hill work: Stride out 5 min. Walk 2 min. Stride out 10 min. Walk 5 min.	Rest.	Walk 15 min. Stride out 10 min. Walk 5 min.	Rolling hill work: Stride out 30 min.
3 EASY	Rest.	Rolling hill work: Stride out 15 min. Walk 5 min.	Rolling hill work: Walk 15 min. Stride out 10 min. Walk 5 min.	Rolling hill work: Stride out 5 min. Walk 2 min. Stride out 5 min. Walk 5 min.	Rest.	Walk 20 min. Stride out 5 min. Walk 5 min.	Rolling hill work: Stride out 30 min.
4 HARD	Rest.	Rolling hill work: Stride out 20 min. Walk 5 min.	Rolling hill work: Walk 15 min. Stride out 10 min. Walk 5 min.	Rolling hill work: Stride out 5 min. Walk 2 min. Stride out 7 min. Walk 5 min.	Rest.	Walk 20 min. Stride out 10 min. Walk 5 min.	Rolling hill work: Stride out 30 min.
5 EASY	Rest.	Rolling hill work: Stride out 20 min. Walk 5 min.	Rolling hill work: Walk 15 min. Stride out 10 min. Walk 5 min.	Rolling hill work: Stride out 5 min. Walk 2 min. Stride out 7 min. Walk 5 min.	Rest.	Walk 20 min. Stride out 10 min. Walk 5 min.	Rolling hill work: Stride out 35 min.
6 HARD	Rest.	Rolling hill work: Stride out 25 min. Walk 5 min.	Rest.	Rolling hill work: Stride out 10 min. Walk 2 min. Stride out 10 min. Walk 5 min.	Rest.	Walk 30 min.	Rolling hill work: Stride out 35 min.

RACEWALKING INTERMEDIATE 8. Achieving Mastery

DAY	1	Strength Work 2	3	Strength Work 4	5	Strength Work 6	7
WEEK 1 EASY	Rest.	Rolling hill work: Stride out 35 min.	Rolling hill work: Walk 5 min. Stride out 5 min. Walk 5 min. Stride out 7 min. Walk 5 min.	Rolling hill work: Walk 10 min. Stride out 10 min. Walk 10 min.	Rest.	Walk 15 min. Stride out 10 min. Walk 2 min.	Rolling hill work: Stride out 35 min. Walk 5 min.
2 MODERATE	Rest.	Rolling hill work: Stride out 35 min.	Rolling hill work: Walk 5 min. Stride out 10 min. Walk 5 min. Stride out 7 min. Walk 5 min.	Rolling hill work: Stride out 25 min. Walk 5 min.	Rest.	Walk 20 min. Stride out 10 min. Walk 2 min.	Rolling hill work: Stride out 35 min. Walk 5 min.
3 EASY	Rest.	Rolling hill work: Stride out 35 min.	Rest.	Rolling hill work: Stride out 20 min. Walk 5 min.	Rest.	Walk 15 min. Stride out 10 min. Walk 2 min.	Rolling hill work: Stride out 35 min. Walk 5 min.
4 HARD	Rest.	Rolling hill work: Stride out 35 min.	Rolling hill work: Stride out 20 min. Walk 5 min.	Rolling hill work: Stride out 25 min. Walk 5 min.	Rest.	Walk 10 min. Stride out 20 min. Walk 2 min.	Rolling hill work: Stride out 35 min. Walk 5 min.
5 EASY							
6 HARD							

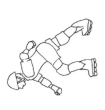

RACEWALKING ADVANCED *9. Awakening the Body*

DAY	1	Strength Work 2	3	Strength Work 4	5	Strength Work 6	7
WEEK **1** EASY	Rest.	Rolling hill work: Stride out 25 min. Walk 5 min.	Walk 10 min. Stride out 20 min. Walk 5 min.	Walk 5 min. Stride out 15 min. Walk 10 min.	Rest.	Walk 20 min. Stride out 20 min. Walk 5 min.	Rolling hill work: Stride out 45 min. Walk 5 min.
2 MODERATE	Rest.	Rolling hill work: Stride out 30 min. Walk 5 min.	Rest.	Rolling hill work: Stride out 25 min. Walk 5 min.	Rest.	Walk 40 min.	Rolling hill work: Stride out 45 min. Walk 5 min.
3 EASY							
4 HARD							
5 EASY							
6 HARD							

DAY / WEEK	1	Strength Work 2	3	4	5	Strength Work 6	7
1 EASY	Rest.	Rolling hill work: Stride out 35 min. Walk 5 min.	Rolling hill work: Walk 5 min. Stride out 30 min. Walk 5 min.	Stride out 15 min. Pick up your pace 10 min. Stride out 5 min.	Rest.	Walk 20 min. Stride out 20 min.	Rolling hill work: Stride out 40 min. Walk 5 min.
2 MODERATE	Rest.	Rolling hill work: Stride out 35 min. Walk 5 min.	Rolling hill work: Walk 5 min. Stride out 40 min. Walk 5 min.	Stride out 20 min. Pick up your pace 10 min. Stride out 5 min.	Rest.	Stride out 40 min.	Rolling hill work: Stride out 40 min. Walk 5 min.
3 EASY	Rest.	Rolling hill work: Stride out 35 min. Walk 5 min.	Rest.	Stride out 20 min. Pick up your pace 10 min. Stride out 5 min.	Rest.	Walk 20 min. Stride out 30 min.	Rolling hill work: Stride out 40 min. Walk 5 min.
4 HARD	Rest.	Rolling hill work: Stride out 35 min. Walk 5 min.	Rolling hill work: Walk 5 min. Stride out 40 min. Walk 5 min.	Stride out 25 min. Pick up your pace 15 min. Stride out 5 min.	Rest.	Walk 10 min. Stride out 20 min.	Rolling hill work: Stride out 40 min. Walk 5 min.
5 EASY	Rest.	Rolling hill work: Stride out 35 min. Walk 5 min.	Game Day.	Walk 20 min. Stride out 20 min.	Rest.	Walk 20 min. Stride out 20 min.	Rolling hill work: Stride out 40 min. Walk 5 min.
6 HARD	Rest.	Rolling hill work: Stride out 35 min. Walk 5 min.	Game Day.	Walk 15 min. Stride out 30 min.	Rest.	Walk 20 min. Stride out 20 min.	Rolling hill work: Stride out 40 min. Walk 5 min.

RACEWALKING ADVANCED   *10. Laying the Foundation*

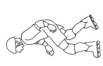

DAY	1	Strength Work 2	3	Strength Work 4	5	Strength Work 6	7
WEEK 1 EASY	Rest.	Stride out 35 min. Keep a steady pace.	Game Day.	Walk 10 min. Stride out 30 min. Walk 5 min.	Rest.	Walk 20 min. Stride out 20 min.	Stride out 45 min. Keep a steady pace.
2 MODERATE	Rest.	Stride out 40 min. Keep a steady pace.	Game Day.	Walk 5 min. Stride out 40 min. Walk 5 min.	Rest.	Walk 20 min. Stride out 20 min.	Stride out 45 min. Keep a steady pace.
3 EASY	Rest.	Stride out 35 min. Keep a steady pace.	Game Day.	Stride out 45 min. Walk 5 min.	Rest.	Walk 20 min. Stride out 20 min.	Stride out 45 min. Keep a steady pace.
4 HARD	Rest.	Stride out 45 min. Keep a steady pace.	Game Day.	Stride out 45 min. Walk 5 min.	Rest.	Walk 20 min. Stride out 20 min.	Stride out 50 min. Keep a steady pace.
5 EASY	Rest.	Walk 5 min. Stride out 15 min. Walk 5 min. Stride out 15 min. Walk 5 min.	Stride out 40 min. Keep a steady pace.	Game Day.	Rest.	Stride out 30 min. Keep a steady pace.	Stride out 45 min. Keep a steady pace.
6 HARD	Rest.	Walk 5 min. Stride out 20 min. Walk 5 min. Stride out 20 min. Walk 5 min.	Stride out 45 min. Keep a steady pace.	Game Day.	Rest.	Stride out 30 min. Keep a steady pace.	Stride out 50 min. Keep a steady pace.

RACEWALKING ADVANCED   *11. Building Endurance*

RACEWALKING ADVANCED   12. Achieving Mastery

DAY	1	Strength Work 2	3	Strength Work 4	5	Strength Work 6	7
WEEK 1 EASY	Rest.	Walk 5 min. Stride out 20 min. Walk 5 min. Stride out 10 min. Walk 5 min.	Stride out 40 min.	Game Day.	Rest.	Stride out 30 min.	Stride out 45 min. Pick up the pace.
2 MODERATE	Rest.	Walk 5 min. Stride out 25 min. Walk 5 min. Stride out 5 min. Walk 5 min.	Stride out 50 min.	Game Day.	Rest.	Stride out 30 min.	Stride out 55 min. Pick up the pace.
3 EASY	Rest.	Walk 5 min. Stride out 35 min. Walk 10 min.	Stride out 30 min.	Game Day.	Rest.	Stride out 30 min.	Stride out 55 min. Pick up the pace.
4 HARD	Rest.	Stride out 35 min.	Stride out 40 min.	Stride out 30 min.	Rest.	Stride out 30 min.	Stride out 60 min. Pick up the pace.
5 EASY							
6 HARD							

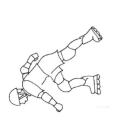

RUNNING

See art, pages 101–127.

TECHNIQUE AND FORM

Running begins as walking. Left. Right. Left. Right. Arms swing loosely at your side with elbows slightly flexed and hands relaxed. Head up. Back straight. Abdomen tight. As you accelerate, eventually you move so fast that you automatically advance to an airborne phase with both feet off the ground at the same time. This single moment expresses the basic difference between walking and running. Running is not a matter of reaching forward to plant each leg and pull your torso to and over it with each step. Actually, the power to thrust each leg forward comes from behind, initiating in your glutes. As the large glute muscle is fired, the leg is swung forward in a surprisingly relaxed biomechanical maneuver. Of course, this relaxation ends in a split second, because in running, your body has much to do. Running is a miracle in shock absorption and energy transfer. When the heel on your extending foot strikes the ground, and you pass your torso over top of it, your foot begins to "load," or take your weight. Your shin (tibia) rotates slightly to the inside. Your loading foot (at first in supination or inversion with ankle angled, pointing the sole of the foot to the inside) flattens under the pressure of your weight, and then, when it has reached its maximum compression (now in pronation or eversion with ankle angled, pointing the sole of the foot to the outside), tendons and muscles recoil like a spring to restore your foot to its neutral position, giving you a boost up and forward. You can also picture your arch flattening out, then springing back into shape, as you roll your weight from your heel onto the ball of your foot. Experts describe this as "vertical-to-longitudinal torque conversion." While your loading foot is doing its work, your rear foot is coming up and around in a cyclical pattern to take its place. But your glutes, legs, and feet aren't working alone. Your arms are pumping in opposition to your foot strikes: left arm for amplifying and transferring energy to the right leg, right arm for amplifying and transferring energy to your left leg. Indeed, running engages the entire body and all major muscle groups.

EQUIPMENT YOU'LL NEED

A watch

A bottle of water

An identification card to put into your pocket

Cell phone (perhaps in a fanny pack)

WHAT TO WEAR

In warm weather, wear shorts and a T-shirt or singlet. Make sure they're made of lightweight material designed to keep you cool and wick sweat away from your body. Additionally, they should be loose enough to be comfortable but snug enough to avoid rubbing and blistering. By the way, if you have trouble with clothing that rubs, wear it inside out so the seams are away from your skin. With T-shirts, you might try chopping away the sleeves and neckline, eliminating the offending seams. You'll make a ragged, no-nonsense fashion statement that will intimidate everyone else at the track.

In cool weather, you can wear running tights under your shorts, or eliminate the shorts completely and go with the tights alone. If it's really cold outside, layering is always best. In extreme weather, you can add long pants that are specifically designed for runners and are made to insulate you from the cold and wick sweat away. They have zippers at the bottom of each leg so you can put them on and get them off easily over your shoes. They're loose enough so you can move, but fitted and soft to keep from rubbing. Keep the T-shirt or singlet, but cover it with a long-sleeved T-shirt, sweatshirt, or weatherproof jacket that can be removed and tied around your waist if you get too hot. Wear a snugly fitting knit hat that you can pull down over your ears. Wear cotton gloves, or gloves made from silk or polypropylene that will wick sweat away from your skin. If you don't have gloves, wear a pair of tube socks over your hands.

Shoes: You need the best pair of running shoes you can afford. Shoes vary widely, as they are specifically engineered to compensate for different surface and distance requirements, body weights, and imbalance problems. When you shop for shoes, take along a pair of socks like the ones you intend to wear when you run. Also, experts suggest that you try on the shoes at the same time of day you intend to work out, because the size of your foot may vary by as much as half a size during the course of your day. When you find a pair of shoes you like, try on *both* shoes. Lace them fully, and run around the sales floor. Make sure you can get off the carpet and onto a hard surface if you really want to get a feel for how they'll perform for you in "real life"—unless you plan to run only on carpet when you train. (We favor one athletic shoe store that allows us to wear the shoes outside on a clean sidewalk they maintain for this purpose.) Put the shoes through their paces—slow, fast, left turn, right turn, pivot, and about-face. Try on more than one pair and test each equally. Pay attention to raised surfaces, seams, and rough spots inside the shoe. They might seem like petty annoyances in the shoe store, but they'll turn into big problems when you start adding on the miles. Avoid being swayed by a shoe's appearance. It's what's inside and underneath that counts. In fact, we ask our clients to evaluate shoes with their eyes closed for at least a moment. In making your final decision about which shoes to buy, remember that comfort and fit are much more important than a fancy sales pitch from a clerk who may or may not be particularly knowledgeable about shoes and the biomechanics of running. *You* take charge here. After all, you're going to be working out in the shoes.

Socks: Socks are optional, but most people enjoy wearing them. They add a layer of protection between your foot and the inside of the shoe. Look for a smooth, snug fit that's free from wrinkles and inside seams. Because even the best socks are an inexpensive investment, go first-class. Purchase athletes' socks that are engineered to wick moisture, or absorb sweat, away from your foot and provide you with a dryer shoe interior, which will help prevent blistering, skin irritations, and odor. Treat yourself to a clean pair of socks with every workout.

Undergarments: Running is a tough sport that places huge demands on the body. Both men and women should wear undergarments that support and protect delicate tissues.

BOREDOM BUSTERS

Listen to music: Portable CD and tape players, and radios with lightweight headsets, are popular among runners. Just make sure that your choice of music is compatible with your planned workout. You know what we mean. Nothing trashes a good pace faster than an operatic funeral dirge. If you're running in the company of other people who are trying to pace their own workouts, be sure you're using a headset that affords you complete privacy. In other words, do everything possible to keep from imposing (or inflicting) your choice of music—and its accompanying rhythms—on other runners. When using a headset, leave one ear totally free so that you can hear what's going on around you and stay alert to your environment. If you're running beside a roadway, leave free the ear that is closest to traffic. Digital stereo is great, but it's dangerous in a workout.

Recruit a partner: For athletes who train outside on streets or on tracks, there's safety in numbers. There's also motivation. You and a friend can work together to keep your training schedules on track. Better yet, join a club or a running group where you can work out with other runners.

Sign up for a race: Nothing motivates a runner like an upcoming competition. Targeting a specific goal on a specific date puts focus and excitement into even the most anemic program. And there's nothing like a souvenir T-shirt for spicing up your wardrobe like a veteran. Many competitions help raise money for charities.

Play utility poles: This game can introduce speed work, or "tempo," into your training. Utility poles are good gauges of precise distance because they are evenly placed beside the road. Pick up your pace from the first pole to the second, then back off until you reach the third pole. Step up your pace again, and so on and so on. As you develop stamina, try increasing the numbers of poles between which you pick up your pace, such as picking up the pace for three poles, then backing off for one pole.

Urban touring: This game for city dwellers was developed by Phil, who trains intensely in New York. The only requirements are city sidewalks and traffic lights. The point of the game is to travel as far as you can without stopping. Run straight down the sidewalk. When you inevitably encounter a stoplight that could impede you from continuing your route, don't stop. Immediately change direction. Run either right or left, following the "Walk" signal. Look both ways first, and continue straight along that route until you encounter another stoplight. Don't stop, change direction. You'll never be sure where you'll travel, and you'll have to make some quick decisions that will take you on an undetermined, random journey. (Phil notes that the game becomes really challenging when you decide it's time to get home.)

TAKING IT TO THE GYM

Indoor track
Treadmill
Elliptical trainer
Stair stepper (in moderation . . .)

INJURY ALERT

Running, in spite of all its benefits, is also a sport in which injuries are common. It is, of course, a repetitive activity. Running causes your feet to hit the ground at forces one and a half to five times your present body weight, and each foot hits the ground a hundred times per mile and over five thousand times per hour. Sports medicine experts classify runners' injuries into two categories: those that are caused by circumstances and those that are caused by the

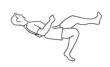

runner's physiology. Of those that are caused by circumstances, training mistakes—running too much, too soon, and too often—lead the list. Of those injuries caused by a runner's physiology, imbalance, misalignment, and inflexibility are the most common. No matter what the cause of the problem, running tends to be fairly unforgiving. Small things make big differences when they're multiplied and amplified to the extent that running demands. Everything has to work. And, equally important, everything has to work together. Breakdowns can occur in perfectly healthy places when the failure is actually somewhere else up or down the line. For example, a weak hamstring that cannot do its job might force compensations all the way down the leg, and show up as pain and dysfunction in the Achilles tendon—nearly forty inches below the real problem. A weakened lower back may caused a slight pelvic list on one side that will drop one leg low and cause the foot to hit the ground a nanosecond before it should. The result could be knee and ankle pain, and a slight limp. The runner might conclude that he has a leg-length discrepancy and slip a lift into the heel of the other shoe. Now the imbalance is even greater and triggers a domino effect of cascading injuries. In running, as in all repetitive activities, preventing an injury requires vigilance and intelligence. So does healing.

TIPS FROM THE EXPERTS

You need to supplement your running program with strength training—particularly for upper body—and flexibility work to offset the hammering and limited range of motion your body takes in the repetitive, forward tracking of a running gait. Pay attention to your body. Buy the best shoes you can afford and select them under the guidance of an experienced, trusted person. Start your running program slowly, then gradually increase your mileage and the intensity of your workouts. If injury strikes, seek advice from a physician who treats runners and running injuries. And once you get that advice, heed it. Be smart and you'll live to run another day.

Please remember to hydrate. Running is a strenuous, demanding sport both in training and competition. Even slight dehydration lowers the circulating volume of blood and causes the core temperature to rise. Symptoms of progressive dehydration include fatigue, lack of coordination, muscle pain and cramping, headache, light-headedness, confusion, disorientation, and fainting. Under extreme circumstances, death can occur. If you feel thirsty, you're already on your way to trouble. Drink early—before thirst sets in—and often. Experts say that water is perfect for short events, but a commercial sport fluid-replacement drink is preferable for events of more than ninety minutes in duration. With either choice, *cold* is best. We want you to play it cool. Drink.

COMING TO TERMS WITH THE TERMS WE USE IN OUR SCHEDULE

Walk: Because running is so hard on the body, we start your program off with some walking to get you used to being on your feet for sustained periods of time before we make more difficult demands.

Jog: This is running at a leisurely, conversational pace. You should be in the minimum range of your target heart rate. We want you to concentrate on perfect form and get used to your shoes.

Run: This is a quickened pace, but still (almost) conversational. You should be in the middle to upper-middle range of your target heart rate.

Pick up the pace: This is race pace. You'll be exerting effort. You should be in the higher ranges of your target heart rate.

Keep a steady pace: Sustain your effort and refrain from speeding up or slowing down.

Surfaces: If we specify the topography (such as rolling hills or flat surfaces), do your best to follow our suggestions. If working out on specific surfaces isn't possible, any surface will do. If we haven't specified a surface, choose one you like.

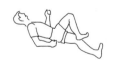

DAY	1	Strength Work 2	3	Strength Work 4	5	Strength Work 6	7
WEEK 1 EASY	Make sure your shoes and clothing are in order.	Walk 15 min. on flat surface.	Walk 15 min. on flat surface.	Walk 15 min. at brisk pace.	Rest.	Walk 5 min. at normal pace. Walk 15 min. at brisk pace.	Walk 5 min. at normal pace. Walk 15 min. at brisk pace.
2 MODERATE	Rest.	Walk 5 min. Jog 5 min. (Easy does it!) Walk 5 min.	Walk 15 min. at moderate pace.	Rest.	Walk 5 min. Jog 5 min. (Easy does it!) Walk 5 min.	Rest.	Walk 5 min. Jog 5 min. (Easy does it!) Walk 5 min.
3 EASY							
4 HARD							
5 EASY							
6 HARD							

RUNNING BEGINNER 1. *Awakening the Body*

RUNNING BEGINNER 2. Laying the Foundation

DAY / WEEK	1	2 (Strength Work)	3	4 (Strength Work)	5	6 (Strength Work)	7
1 EASY	Rest.	Walk 20 min.	Walk 5 min. Jog/Walk 20 min. (alternate jogging and walking in 5-min. intervals). Walk 5 min.	Walk 20 min.	Rest.	Walk 20 min.	Walk 5 min. Jog/Walk 10 min. (alternate jogging and walking in 1-min. intervals). Walk 5 min.
2 MODERATE	Rest.	Walk 10 min. Jog 20 min. Walk 10 min.	Walk 20 min. on flat surface.	Rest.	Walk 5 min. Jog/Walk 10 min. (alternate jogging and walking in 1-min. intervals). Walk 5 min.	Rest.	Walk 10 min. Jog 5 min. Walk 10 min.
3 EASY	Rest.	Walk 25 min. on flat surface.	Rest.	Walk 25 min. at brisk pace.	Rest.	Walk 20 min. at brisk pace.	Walk 5 min. Jog 5 min. Walk 5 min. Jog 5 min. Walk 5 min.
4 HARD	Rest.	Walk 5 min. Jog 5 min. Walk 5 min. Jog 5 min.	Walk 25 min. at brisk pace. Walk 5 min. at easy pace.	Walk 5 min. at brisk pace. Jog 5 min. Walk 5 min. at easy pace.	Rest.	Walk 20 min. at brisk pace.	Hill walk: Uphill for 15 min. Downhill for 15 min.
5 EASY	Rest.	Walk 5 min. Jog 10 min. Walk 5 min. Jog 5 min.	Rest.	Rest.	Walk 5 min. Jog/Walk 10 min. (alternate jogging and walking in 1-min. intervals). Walk 10 min.	Rest.	Walk 5 min. Jog 10 min. Walk 10 min.
6 HARD	Rest.	Hill walk at brisk pace: Uphill for 15 min. Downhill for 15 min.	Walk 5 min. Jog 15 min. Walk 5 min.	Walk 10 min. at easy pace. Jog 5 min. Walk 10 min. at brisk pace.	Rest.	Walk 20 min. at brisk pace on flat surface.	Walk 5 min. Jog 10 min. Walk 10 min.

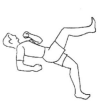

DAY	1	Strength Work 2	3	Strength Work 4	5	Strength Work 6	7
WEEK 1 EASY	Rest.	Rolling hill work: Walk 5 min. Jog 5 min. Walk 5 min. Jog 5 min. Walk 5 min.	Walk 5 min. Jog 10 min. Walk 5 min.	Rest.	Rolling hill work: Walk 5 min. Jog 10 min. Walk 5 min. Jog 5 min. Walk 5 min.	Rest.	Walk 5 min. Jog 20 min. Walk 5 min.
2 MODERATE	Rest.	Rolling hill work: Walk 5 min. Jog 10 min. Walk 5 min. Jog 5 min. Walk 5 min.	Jog 5 min. Run 10 min. Jog 5 min.	Walk 10 min. Run 10 min. Walk 10 min.	Rest.	Walk 5 min. Jog 15 min. Walk 10 min.	Walk 5 min. Jog 20 min. Walk 5 min.
3 EASY	Rest.	Rolling hill work: Walk 5 min. Jog 10 min. Walk 5 min. Jog 10 min. Walk 5 min.	Jog 5 min. Run 15 min. Jog 5 min.	Rest.	Rolling hill work: Walk 15 min. Jog 15 min. Walk 10 min.	Rest.	Jog 15 min. Run 20 min. Jog 5 min.
4 HARD	Rest.	Rolling hill work: Walk 5 min. Jog 10 min. Walk 5 min. Jog 20 min. Walk 5 min.	Jog 5 min. Run 15 min. Jog 5 min.	Rolling hill work: Walk 5 min. Jog 5 min. Walk 5 min. Jog 10 min. Walk 5 min.	Rest.	Walk 5 min. Jog 20 min. Walk 5 min. Jog 5 min. Walk 5 min.	Jog 15 min. Run 25 min. Jog 5 min.
5 EASY	Rest.	Rolling hill work: Walk 5 min. Jog 15 min. Walk 5 min. Jog 10 min. Walk 5 min.	Jog 5 min. Run 20 min. Jog 5 min.	Rest.	Rolling hill work: Walk 5 min. Jog 10 min. Walk 5 min. Jog 5 min. Walk 5 min.	Rest.	Jog 25 min.
6 HARD	Rest.	Rolling hill work: Walk 5 min. Jog 10 min. Walk 5 min. Jog 15 min. Walk 5 min.	Walk 5 min. Run 25 min. Walk 5 min.	Walk 5 min. Jog 5 min. Walk 5 min. Jog 20 min. Walk 5 min.	Rest.	Jog 5 min. Run 10 min. Jog 5 min.	Jog 30 min.

RUNNING BEGINNER *3. Building Endurance*

RUNNING BEGINNER 4. Achieving Mastery

DAY	1	Strength Work 2	3	Strength Work 4	5	Strength Work 6	7
WEEK 1 EASY	Rest.	Rolling hill work: Jog 5 min. Run 25 min. Jog 5 min.	Jog 5 min. Run 15 min. Jog 5 min. Run 10 min. Jog 5 min.	Rest.	Rolling hill work: Jog 5 min. Run 5 min. Jog 5 min. Repeat entire pattern.	Jog 5 min. Run 20 min. Jog 5 min.	Jog 5 min. Run 25 min. Jog 5 min.
2 MODERATE	Rest.	Rolling hill work: Jog 5 min. Run 25 min. Jog 5 min.	Jog 5 min. Run 10 min. Jog 5 min. Run 10 min. Jog 5 min.	Rolling hill work: Jog 5 min. Run 15 min. Jog 5 min. Run 10 min. Jog 5 min.	Rest.	Rolling hill work: Jog 10 min. Run 15 min. Jog 5 min.	Jog 20 min. Run 10 min. Jog 10 min.
3 EASY							
4 HARD							
5 EASY							
6 HARD							

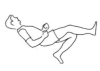

DAY	1	Strength Work 2	3	Strength Work 4	5	Strength Work 6	7
WEEK 1 EASY	Rest.	On flat surface: Jog 5 min. Run 25 min. Jog 5 min.	Jog 5 min. Run 10 min. Jog 5 min. Run 10 min. Jog 5 min.	Rolling hill work: Jog 5 min. Run 15 min. Jog 5 min. Run 10 min. Jog 5 min.	Rest.	Rolling hill work: Jog 10 min. Run 15 min. Jog 5 min.	Rolling hill work: Jog 20 min. Run 10 min. Jog 10 min.
2 MODERATE	Rest.	Rolling hill work: Jog 10 min. Run 25 min. Jog 10 min.	Jog 5 min. Run 15 min. Jog 5 min. Run 15 min. Jog 5 min.	Rolling hill work: Jog 10 min. For 30 min., alternate 1 min. running with 1 min. jogging. Jog 5 min.	Rest.	Rolling hill work: Jog 10 min. Run 20 min. Jog 5 min.	Hill work: Run uphill 20 min. Run downhill 15 min.
3 EASY							
4 HARD							
5 EASY							
6 HARD							

RUNNING INTERMEDIATE   6. Laying the Foundation

DAY	1	Strength Work 2	3	Strength Work 4	5	Strength Work 6	7
WEEK 1 EASY	Rest.	Rolling hill work: Jog 30 min.	Jog 5 min. Run 15 min. Jog 15 min. Run 15 min. Jog 5 min.	Rolling hill work: Jog 10 min. For 25 min., alternate 1 min. jogging with 1 min. running. Jog 5 min.	Rest.	Rolling hill work: Jog 10 min. Run 20 min. Jog 5 min.	Hill work: Alternate jogging and running: Uphill 20 min. Downhill 15 min.
2 MODERATE	Rest.	Rolling hill work: Jog 20 min. Run 10 min. Jog 5 min.	On flat surface: Jog 5 min. Run 20 min. Jog 5 min. Run 10 min. Jog 5 min.	Rolling hill work: Jog 5 min. For 35 min., alternate 5 min. jogging with 5 min. running. Jog 5 min.	Rest.	Rolling hill work: Jog 5 min. Run 25 min. Jog 5 min.	Hill work: Alternate jogging and running: Uphill 25 min. Downhill 20 min.
3 EASY	Rest.	Rolling hill work: Jog 15 min. Run 10 min. Jog 5 min.	Jog 5 min. Run 15 min. Jog 5 min. Run 10 min. Jog 5 min.	Rolling hill work: Jog 5 min. For 35 min., alternate 5 min. jogging with 5 min. running. Jog 5 min.	Rest.	Rolling hill work: Jog 35 min.	Hill work: Alternate jogging and running: Uphill 25 min. Downhill 20 min.
4 HARD	Rest.	Rolling hill work: Jog 30 min. Run 15 min. Jog 5 min.	Jog 5 min. Run 20 min. Jog 5 min. Run 10 min. Jog 5 min.	Rolling hill work: Jog 5 min. For 35 min., alternate 1 min. jogging with 1 min. running. Jog 5 min.	Rest.	Rolling hill work: Run 25 min. Jog 5 min.	Hill work: Alternate jogging and running: Uphill 25 min. Downhill 20 min.
5 EASY	Rest.	Rolling hill work: Jog 10 min. Run 10 min. Jog 5 min.	Jog 10 min. Run 10 min. Jog 5 min. Run 5 min. Jog 5 min.	Rolling hill work: Jog 5 min. For 35 min., alternate 5 min. jogging with 5 min. running. Jog 5 min.	Rest.	Rolling hill work: Jog 5 min. Run 25 min. Jog 5 min.	Hill work: Alternate jogging and running: Uphill 25 min. Downhill 20 min.
6 HARD	Rest.	Rolling hill work: Jog 10 min. Run 20 min. Jog 5 min.	Jog 10 min. Run 20 min. Jog 5 min. Run 5 min. Jog 5 min.	Rolling hill work: Jog 5 min. For 35 min., alternate 5 min. jogging with 5 min. running. Jog 5 min.	Rest.	Rolling hill work: Run 30 min. Jog 5 min.	Rolling hill work: Jog 10 min. Run 20 min. Jog 5 min. Run 5 min. Jog 5 min.

DAY	1	Strength Work 2	3	Strength Work 4	5	Strength Work 6	7
WEEK 1 EASY	Rest.	Rolling hill work: Run 15 min. Jog 5 min.	Rolling hill work: Jog 10 min. Run 10 min. Jog 5 min.	Rolling hill work: Run 5 min. Jog 2 min. Run 5 min. Jog 5 min.	Rest.	Jog 20 min. Run 5 min. Jog 5 min.	Rolling hill work: Jog 30 min.
2 MODERATE	Rest.	Rolling hill work: Run 15 min. Jog 5 min.	Rolling hill work: Jog 10 min. Run 10 min. Jog 5 min.	Rolling hill work: Run 5 min. Jog 2 min. Run 10 min. Jog 5 min.	Rest.	Jog 15 min. Run 10 min. Jog 5 min.	Rolling hill work: Run 30 min.
3 EASY	Rest.	Rolling hill work: Run 15 min. Jog 5 min.	Rolling hill work: Jog 15 min. Run 10 min. Jog 5 min.	Rolling hill work: Run 5 min. Jog 2 min. Run 5 min. Jog 5 min.	Rest.	Jog 20 min. Run 5 min. Jog 5 min.	Rolling hill work: Run 30 min.
4 HARD	Rest.	Rolling hill work: Run 20 min. Jog 5 min.	Rolling hill work: Jog 15 min. Run 10 min. Jog 5 min.	Rolling hill work: Run 5 min. Jog 2 min. Run 7 min. Jog 5 min.	Rest.	Jog 20 min. Run 10 min. Jog 5 min.	Rolling hill work: Run 30 min.
5 EASY	Rest.	Rolling hill work: Run 20 min. Jog 5 min.	Rolling hill work: Jog 15 min. Run 10 min. Jog 5 min.	Rolling hill work: Run 5 min. Jog 2 min. Run 7 min. Jog 5 min.	Rest.	Jog 20 min. Run 10 min. Jog 5 min.	Rolling hill work: Run 35 min.
6 HARD	Rest.	Rolling hill work: Run 25 min. Jog 5 min.	Rest.	Rolling hill work: Run 10 min. Jog 2 min. Run 10 min. Jog 5 min.	Rest.	Jog 30 min.	Rolling hill work: Run 35 min.

RUNNING INTERMEDIATE *7. Building Endurance*

RUNNING INTERMEDIATE 8. Achieving Mastery

DAY	1	Strength Work 2	3	Strength Work 4	5	Strength Work 6	7
WEEK 1 EASY	Rest.	Rolling hill work: Run 35 min.	Rolling hill work: Jog 5 min. Run 5 min. Run 7 min. Jog 5 min.	Rolling hill work: Jog 10 min. Run 10 min. Jog 10 min.	Rest.	Jog 15 min. Run 10 min. Jog 2 min.	Rolling hill work: Run 35 min. Jog 5 min.
2 MODERATE	Rest.	Rolling hill work: Run 35 min.	Rolling hill work: Jog 5 min. Run 10 min. Run 5 min. Run 7 min. Jog 5 min.	Rolling hill work: Run 25 min. Jog 5 min.	Rest.	Jog 20 min. Run 10 min. Jog 2 min.	Rolling hill work: Run 35 min. Jog 5 min.
3 EASY	Rest.	Rolling hill work: Run 35 min.	Rest.	Rolling hill work: Run 20 min. Jog 5 min.	Rest.	Jog 15 min. Run 10 min. Jog 2 min.	Rolling hill work: Run 35 min. Jog 5 min.
4 HARD	Rest.	Rolling hill work: Run 35 min.	Rolling hill work: Run 20 min. Jog 5 min.	Rolling hill work: Run 25 min. Jog 5 min.	Rest.	Jog 10 min. Run 20 min. Jog 2 min.	Rolling hill work: Run 35 min. Jog 5 min.
5 EASY							
6 HARD							

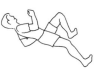

DAY	1	Strength Work 2	3	Strength Work 4	5	Strength Work 6	7
WEEK 1 EASY	Rest.	Rolling hill work: Run 25 min. Jog 5 min.	Jog 10 min. Run 20 min. Jog 5 min.	Jog 5 min. Run 15 min. Jog 10 min.	Rest.	Jog 20 min. Run 20 min. Jog 5 min.	Rolling hill work: Run 45 min. Jog 5 min.
2 MODERATE	Rest.	Rolling hill work: Run 30 min. Jog 5 min.	Rest.	Rolling hill work: Run 25 min. Jog 5 min.	Rest.	Jog 40 min.	Rolling hill work: Run 45 min. Jog 5 min.
3 EASY							
4 HARD							
5 EASY							
6 HARD							

RUNNING ADVANCED   9. Awakening the Body

RUNNING ADVANCED   10. Laying the Foundation

WEEK	DAY 1	Strength Work / DAY 2	DAY 3	Strength Work / DAY 4	DAY 5	Strength Work / DAY 6	DAY 7
1 EASY	Rest.	Rolling hill work: Run 35 min. Jog 5 min.	Rolling hill work: Jog 5 min. Run 30 min. Jog 5 min.	Run 15 min. Pick up your pace 10 min. Run 5 min.	Rest.	Jog 20 min. Run 20 min.	Rolling hill work: Run 40 min. Jog 5 min.
2 MODERATE	Rest.	Rolling hill work: Run 35 min. Jog 5 min.	Rolling hill work: Jog 5 min. Run 40 min. Jog 5 min.	Run 20 min. Pick up your pace 10 min. Run 5 min.	Rest.	Run 40 min.	Rolling hill work: Run 40 min. Jog 5 min.
3 EASY	Rest.	Rolling hill work: Run 35 min. Jog 5 min.	Rest.	Run 20 min. Pick up your pace 10 min. Run 5 min.	Rest.	Jog 20 min. Run 30 min.	Rolling hill work: Run 40 min. Jog 5 min.
4 HARD	Rest.	Rolling hill work: Run 35 min. Jog 5 min.	Rolling hill work: Jog 5 min. Run 40 min. Jog 5 min.	Run 25 min. Pick up your pace 15 min. Run 5 min.	Rest.	Jog 10 min. Run 20 min.	Rolling hill work: Run 40 min. Jog 5 min.
5 EASY	Rest.	Rolling hill work: Run 35 min. Jog 5 min.	Game Day.	Jog 20 min. Run 20 min.	Rest.	Jog 20 min. Run 20 min.	Rolling hill work: Run 40 min. Jog 5 min.
6 HARD	Rest.	Rolling hill work: Run 35 min. Jog 5 min.	Game Day.	Jog 15 min. Run 30 min.	Rest.	Jog 20 min. Run 20 min.	Rolling hill work: Run 40 min. Jog 5 min.

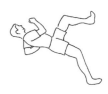

RUNNING ADVANCED   *11. Building Endurance*

DAY / WEEK	1	Strength Work 2	3	Strength Work 4	5	Strength Work 6	7
1 EASY	Rest.	Run 35 min. Keep a steady pace.	Game Day.	Jog 10 min. Run 30 min. Jog 5 min.	Rest.	Jog 20 min. Run 20 min.	Run 45 min. Keep a steady pace.
2 MODERATE	Rest.	Run 40 min. Keep a steady pace.	Game Day.	Jog 5 min. Run 40 min. Jog 5 min.	Rest.	Jog 20 min. Run 20 min.	Run 45 min. Keep a steady pace.
3 EASY	Rest.	Run 35 min. Keep a steady pace.	Game Day.	Run 45 min. Jog 5 min.	Rest.	Jog 20 min. Run 20 min.	Run 45 min. Keep a steady pace.
4 HARD	Rest.	Run 45 min. Keep a steady pace.	Game Day.	Run 45 min. Jog 5 min.	Rest.	Jog 20 min. Run 20 min.	Run 50 min. Keep a steady pace.
5 EASY	Rest.	Jog 5 min. Run 15 min. Jog 5 min. Run 15 min. Jog 5 min.	Run 40 min. Keep a steady pace.	Game Day.	Rest.	Run 30 min. Keep a steady pace.	Run 45 min. Keep a steady pace.
6 HARD	Rest.	Jog 5 min. Run 20 min. Jog 5 min. Run 20 min. Jog 5 min.	Run 45 min. Keep a steady pace.	Game Day.	Rest.	Run 30 min. Keep a steady pace.	Run 50 min. Keep a steady pace.

DAY

WEEK	1	Strength Work 2	3	Strength Work 4	5	Strength Work 6	7
1 EASY	Rest.	Jog 5 min. Run 20 min. Jog 5 min. Run 10 min. Jog 5 min.	Run 40 min.	Game Day.	Rest.	Run 30 min.	Run 45 min. Pick up the pace.
2 MODERATE	Rest.	Jog 5 min. Run 25 min. Jog 5 min. Run 5 min. Jog 5 min.	Run 50 min.	Game Day.	Rest.	Run 30 min.	Run 55 min. Pick up the pace.
3 EASY	Rest.	Jog 5 min. Run 35 min. Jog 10 min.	Run 30 min.	Game Day.	Rest.	Run 30 min.	Run 55 min. Pick up the pace.
4 HARD	Rest.	Run 35 min.	Run 40 min.	Run 30 min.	Rest.	Run 30 min.	Run 60 min. Pick up the pace.
5 EASY							
6 HARD							

RUNNING ADVANCED   *12. Achieving Mastery*

10. The Ten Best Cardio-Fit Activities and Training Schedules   **117**

JUMPING ROPE

See art, pages 129–163.

TECHNIQUE AND FORM

Jumping rope is a sport so ancient that we are unable to trace it to its origins. Likely, the first jump rope was invented by a bored cave dweller who ripped down a vine, happily swung it over his head and under his feet, and sang, "Grog and Blork sitting in a tree K-I-S-S-I-N-G!" We'll never know for sure how it all began, but we do know how jumping rope is used today for fun and fitness. We especially like jumping rope because the workout is a good one, and the equipment is inexpensive, easy to find, and fits into a suitcase. Also, the workout is contained. In other words, you don't have to go anywhere to do it, and you don't need a lot of room in which to work out. A few square feet in your living room or hotel room will do nicely. Remember to scoot furniture out of the way, and make sure you have plenty of clearance overhead so you don't accidentally lasso the chandelier with your first jump. The softer the surface (like carpet, or a wooden floor that gives) the easier on your feet and legs. Concrete is very unforgiving. If you like, you can even take your jump rope outside. As with indoors, the softer the outdoor surface, the more jumper-friendly.

Stand up straight with your feet about six inches apart and your knees relaxed. Hold the ends of the rope firmly, one end in each hand. Start with the rope looped behind your back, just touching the backs of your ankles. Relax the tension on the rope, and swing it in an arc behind you and over your head. Pass the rope all the way over the top of your head and bring the bottom of the loop to the floor in front of you. As you continue the arc, hop lightly on your toes. The rope will pass under your feet. This hop is most easily executed if you build a tiny momentum into it. The rhythm is HOP hophop HOP hophop HOP hophop. In your workout schedule, this basic hop is called the *JUMP.* You'll notice that we introduce more advanced footwork—the *SKIP*—when you're more experienced and your body is conditioned to withstand the stresses that jumping will put on your feet, legs, and hips. The *SKIP* is just that: skipping in place. When the rope passes under your feet, jump with one foot. The other should be slightly behind you and raised higher than the jumping foot. As the rope passes under your jumping foot, the foot behind is swung forward to replace the jumping foot. It's complicated to describe, but easy to figure out for anyone who's ever been eight years old. The *SKIP* is dancelike, delivers a harder workout, and requires more balance and coordination.

Don't be deceived by the inevitable associations of jumping rope with little kids. Jumping rope is way beyond child's play. This workout is a staple in the training of many professional athletes, including football and basketball players, and boxers.

EQUIPMENT YOU'LL NEED

A clock or a watch

A bottle of water

An identification card to put into your pocket if you go out

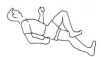

A rope of any diameter: You determine the length by holding one of the two ends of the rope in each hand. Keeping your upper arms and elbows snug with your body, flex your elbows until your lower arms are parallel with the floor. The center point between the two ends (the bottom of the loop you form when you hold the ends and let the rope relax) should touch the floor with about six inches of slack. In other words, as you swing the rope behind you and over your head, the loop should comfortably clear the top of your head. As you bring the loop over your head and to the ground, it should drag very slightly, but not so much that you'll trip. You can take up slack by wrapping the rope around your hands. There are commercial jump ropes available in stores that sell sporting goods and toys, but it's not necessary to get fancy. Almost any rope will do as long as it has a little heft to it and is long enough.

WHAT TO WEAR

Dress so that you'll be comfortable and can move easily. Keep clothing simple and fairly tight-fitting so you won't catch anything in the rope.

Because there is a great deal of ballistic bouncing, you need extra support for all your anatomical parts that are prone to motion. Men and women alike should consider investing in undergarments that are specifically designed for sports. These garments should wick sweat away from your body so you'll keep cool, be free of seams to avoid rubbing a sore spot on delicate skin, and offer you snug support.

The best shoes for jumping rope are those designed for aerobic dancing and cross-training. You'll want a lot of support and cushion under the balls of your feet. Also, select shoes that have good, firm support on the sides, so your ankles will be stable. We recommend socks for extra cushion, blister control, and sweat-wicking.

BOREDOM BUSTERS

Listen to music: Music is always useful for getting and keeping a rhythm. No headsets allowed. You don't want to tangle rope and wire, and macramé yourself into a sweaty wall hanging. Make sure that your choice of music has a good beat. Also, you might have to turn the sound up so that the music is louder than you're accustomed to. From inside your head, your own breathing and the thud-tada-thud-tada-thud of your feet hitting the floor will drown out soft sounds. Turn the music up before you begin the workout so you won't have to stop in the middle to adjust.

Sing: At first you might have difficulty sustaining a long note, because you'll feel out of breath. So what? Enjoy a little Broadway, baby.

Rhyme: One of the real enchantments about jumping rope is the practice of calling cadence, or reciting rhymes that are as much a part of the sport as the rope. Here are a few from your childhood that will remind you that working out is about having fun. (You don't have to sing them out loud; you can just *think* them and still enjoy the silliness.)

I eat my peas with honey.
I've done it all my life.
It makes the peas taste funny,
But keeps them on the knife.
How many peas stick on my knife?
One, two, three . . .

{Girl's name} and {boy's name} sitting in a tree,
K-I-S-S-I-N-G.
First comes love, then comes marriage,
Then comes {friend's name} in a baby carriage!

Lincoln, Lincoln, I've been thinkin',
What on earth have you been drinkin'?
Smells like whiskey, tastes like wine.
Oh my gosh! It's turpentine!

I went downtown to the alligator farm.
I sat on the fence and the fence broke down.
The alligator bit me by the seat of my pants,
And made me do the hula dance.

Travel: We introduce the *SKIP* into your schedule when your body is accustomed to the stresses of the more basic *JUMP.* When we designed the workouts, we intended the *SKIP* to be done in place, but it's possible to move forward rather quickly with this step. If you are feeling adventuresome, you can cover distance as you work out. If you do add mileage to your *SKIP* workout, be careful about the changing topography of the surfaces. We don't want your *SKIP* to become a *SPLAT.*

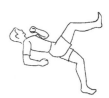

TAKING IT TO THE GYM

There is no substitute equipment with the benefits of jumping rope in the gym, but there's nothing to stop you from taking your own.

INJURY ALERT

Jumping rope, in spite of all its benefits, might very well be the ultimate repetitive activity. For this reason, you're going to have to be vigilant with regard to even small irritations and injuries that are never given time to heal because you're pounding them over and over and over. Little problems don't take long to become big ones. In jumpers, we see trauma to the ball of the foot and irritations from the arch of the foot all the way up through the hip and lower back. Of particular note are shin splints: painful microtears in the connective tissue along the front of the tibia that occur when the leg isn't strong or flexible enough to absorb the shock of the jump on the ball of the foot. Injuries are most commonly caused by jumping too much too soon, and by physical imbalance, misalignment, and inflexibility.

TIPS FROM THE EXPERTS

Be sure to hydrate before, during, and after your workouts. Pay close attention to your posture, so you always jump with good form. Make sure your shoes and socks fit properly. Treat small injuries and irritations immediately, before they get out of hand.

You will want to supplement your jump rope program with strength training—particularly for upper body—and flexibility work to offset the hammering and limited range of motion your body takes in the repetitive tracking of the jump.

COMING TO TERMS WITH THE TERMS OF YOUR SCHEDULE

Jumping jacks: Yep. You read that right. They are your standard old jumping jacks, done without your rope. We use them to get you used to jumping and landing on your feet in rhythm.

Walk: This is just a walk without your rope to get you on your feet and out the door a few times in the first couple of weeks of your program before we start pounding your hips, legs, and feet.

Jump: This is the standard bounce we defined above. It's a leisurely, conversational pace. You should be in the minimum to middle range of your target heart rate.

Skip: Also defined above, this is a quickened pace, but still conversational. You should be in the middle to upper range of your target heart rate.

Double jump: This is passing the rope beneath your feet twice while you're airborne once. It tightens up your upper body and forces you to work a little more quickly and harder. You should be in the higher ranges of your target heart rate.

Repeat × _____: This is a simple instruction that means you should repeat the workout as many times as the number specifies.

Surface: Make sure it's smooth, clear from debris, and has a little "give" to it.

JUMPING ROPE BEGINNER   1. Awakening the Body

	DAY 1	Strength Work 2	3	Strength Work 4	5	Strength Work 6	7
WEEK 1 EASY	Make sure your equipment, shoes, and clothing are in order.	Walk 15 min.	Rest.	Jumping jacks 30 sec. Rest 1 min. Jumping jacks 30 sec. Rest 1 min. Walk 5 min.	Rest.	Walk 5 min. Jump 30 sec. Rest 1 min. Jump 30 sec. Rest 1 min. Walk 5 min.	Walk 15 min.
2 MODERATE	Rest.	Jumping jacks 30 sec. Rest 1 min. Jumping jacks 30 sec. Rest 1 min. Walk 5 min.	Rest.	Walk 5 min. Jump 30 sec. Rest 1 min. Jump 30 sec. Rest 1 min. Walk 5 min.	Rest.	Walk 20 min.	Walk 5 min. Jump 30 sec. Rest 1 min. Jump 30 sec. Rest 1 min. Walk 10 min.
3 EASY							
4 HARD							
5 EASY							
6 HARD							

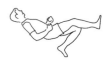

JUMPING ROPE BEGINNER *2. Laying the Foundation*

DAY	1	Strength Work 2	3	Strength Work 4	5	Strength Work 6	7
WEEK 1 EASY	Rest.	Walk 20 min.	Jumping jacks 30 sec. Rest 1 min. Jumping jacks 1 min. Rest 1 min. Jumping jacks 1 min. Walk 10 min.	Walk 5 min. Jump 30 sec. Rest 1 min. (REPEAT × 4) Walk 10 min.	Rest.	Walk 5 min. Jump 30 sec. Rest 1 min. (REPEAT × 4) Walk 10 min.	Walk 20 min.
2 MODERATE	Rest.	Walk 5 min. Jump 30 sec. Rest 1 min. Jump 1 min. Rest 1 min. Walk 10 min.	Jumping jacks 30 sec. Rest 1 min. Jumping jacks 1 min. Rest 1 min. Jumping jacks 1 min. Walk 10 min.	Rest.	Walk 5 min. Jump 30 sec. Rest 1 min. (REPEAT × 4) Walk 10 min.	Rest.	Walk 25 min.
3 EASY	Rest.	Walk 5 min. Jump 30 sec. Rest 1 min. (REPEAT × 4) Walk 10 min.	Rest.	Walk 5 min. Jump 30 sec. Rest 1 min. (REPEAT × 4) Walk 10 min.	Rest.	Walk 5 min. Jump 30 sec. Rest 1 min. (REPEAT × 4) Walk 10 min.	Walk 25 min.
4 HARD	Rest.	Walk 5 min. Jump 1 min. Rest 1 min. (REPEAT × 3) Walk 10 min.	Walk 5 min. Jump 30 sec. Rest 1 min. (REPEAT × 3) Walk 10 min.	Walk 5 min. Jump 1 min. Rest 1 min. (REPEAT × 3) Walk 10 min.	Rest.	Walk 5 min. Jump 2 min. Walk 10 min.	Walk 25 min.
5 EASY	Rest.	Walk 5 min. Jump 2 min. Walk 10 min.	Rest.	Rest.	Walk 5 min. Jump 1 min., 30 sec. Rest 1 min. (REPEAT × 4) Walk 10 min.	Rest.	Walk 5 min. Jump 3 min. Walk 10 min.
6 HARD	Rest.	Walk 5 min. Jump 30 sec. Walk 1 min. (REPEAT × 5) Walk 10 min.	Walk 5 min. Jump 1 min. Walk 1 min. (REPEAT × 3) Walk 10 min.	Walk 5 min. Jump 2 min. Walk 1 min. Jump 2 min. Walk 10 min.	Rest.	Walk 5 min. Jump 30 sec. Walk 30 sec. (REPEAT × 4) Walk 10 min.	Walk 5 min. Jump 4 min. Walk 10 min.

JUMPING ROPE BEGINNER 3. *Building Endurance*

DAY / WEEK	1	2 (Strength Work)	3	4 (Strength Work)	5	6 (Strength Work)	7
1 EASY	Rest.	Walk 5 min. Jump 30 sec. (REPEAT × 5) Walk 5 min.	Walk 5 min. Jump 2 min. Rest 1 min. (REPEAT × 2) Walk 5 min.	Rest.	Walk 5 min. Jump 30 sec. Rest 30 sec. (REPEAT × 6) Walk 5 min.	Rest.	Walk 5 min. Jump 5 min. Walk 5 min.
2 MODERATE	Rest.	Walk 5 min. Jump 3 min. Rest 1 min. (REPEAT × 2) Walk 5 min.	Walk 5 min. Jump 3 min. Rest 1 min. (REPEAT × 2) Walk 5 min.	Walk 5 min. Jump 3 min. Rest 1 min. (REPEAT × 2) Walk 5 min.	Rest.	Walk 5 min. Jump 30 sec. Rest 30 sec. (REPEAT × 6)	Walk 5 min. Jump 6 min. Walk 5 min.
3 EASY	Rest.	Walk 5 min. Jump 3 min. Rest 1 min. (REPEAT × 2) Jump 1 min.	Walk 5 min. Jump 1 min. Rest 1 min. (REPEAT × 5) Walk 5 min.	Rest.	Walk 5 min. Jump 30 sec. Rest 30 sec. (REPEAT × 8)	Rest.	Walk 5 min. Jump 7 min. Walk 5 min.
4 HARD	Rest.	Jump 3 min. Rest 1 min. (REPEAT × 2) Jump 2 min.	Jump 6 min.	Jump 3 min. Rest 1 min. Jump 2 min. Rest 1 min. Jump 1 min.	Rest.	Jump 30 sec. Rest 30 sec. (REPEAT × 6)	Jump 8 min.
5 EASY	Rest.	Jump 4 min. Rest 1 min. Jump 3 min. Rest 1 min. Jump 2 min.	Jump 5 min.	Rest.	Jump 30 sec. Rest 30 sec. (REPEAT × 7)	Rest.	Jump 9 min.
6 HARD	Rest.	Jump 5 min. Rest 1 min. Jump 3 min. Rest 1 min. Jump 2 min.	Jump 7 min.	Jump 4 min. Rest 1 min. Jump 3 min. Rest 1 min. Jump 2 min.	Rest.	Jump 30 sec. Rest 30 sec. (REPEAT × 8)	Jump 10 min.

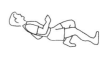

DAY	1	2	3	4	5	6	7
		Strength Work		Strength Work		Strength Work	
WEEK 1 EASY	Rest.	Jump 5 min. Rest 1 min. Jump 4 min. Rest 1 min. Jump 2 min.	Jump 8 min.	Rest.	Jump 30 sec. Rest 30 sec. (REPEAT × 8)	Jump 30 sec. Rest 30 sec. (REPEAT × 5)	Jump 11 min.
2 MODERATE	Rest.	Jump 6 min. Rest 1 min. Jump 6 min.	Jump 9 min.	Jump 1 min. Rest 1 min. (REPEAT × 9)	Rest.	Jump 30 sec. Rest 30 sec. (REPEAT × 6)	Jump 12 min.
3 EASY							
4 HARD							
5 EASY							
6 HARD							

JUMPING ROPE BEGINNER *4. Achieving Mastery*

JUMPING ROPE INTERMEDIATE

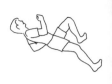

DAY	1	2 Strength Work	3	4 Strength Work	5	6 Strength Work	7
WEEK 1 EASY	Rest.	Jump 6 min.; rest 1. Jump 4 min.; rest 1. Jump 2 min.; rest 1. Jump 1 min.	Jump 6 min.	Jump 7 min.; rest 1. Jump 6 min.	Rest.	Jump 1 min. Rest 1 min. (REPEAT × 10)	Jump 13 min.
2 MODERATE	Rest.	Jump 1 min.; rest 1. Jump 3 min.; rest 1. Jump 5 min.; rest 1. Jump 6 min.	Jump 7 min.	Jump 8 min.; rest 1. Jump 6 min.	Rest.	Jump 20 min. Skip 10 min.	Jump 14 min.
3 EASY							
4 HARD							
5 EASY							
6 HARD							

5. Awakening the Body

DAY WEEK	1	Strength Work 2	3	Strength Work 4	5	Strength Work 6	7
1 EASY	Rest.	Jump 2 min.; rest 1. Jump 6 min.; rest 1. Jump 5 min.; rest 1. Jump 3 min.	Jump 7 min.	Jump 2 min. Rest 1 min. (REPEAT × 4)	Rest.	Jump 1 min. Rest 1 min. (REPEAT × 8)	Jump 14 min.
2 MODERATE	Rest.	Jump 5 min.; rest 1. Jump 6 min.; rest 1. Jump 5 min.	Jump 8 min.	Jump 3 min. Rest 1 min. (REPEAT × 5)	Rest.	Jump 1 min. Rest 1 min. (REPEAT × 9)	Jump 16 min.
3 EASY	Rest.	Jump 4 min.; rest 1. Jump 4 min.; rest 1. Jump 4 min.; rest 1. Jump 4 min.	Jump 8 min.	Jump 2 min. Rest 1 min. (REPEAT × 5)	Rest.	Jump 1 min. Rest 1 min. (REPEAT × 10)	Jump 15 min.
4 HARD	Rest.	Jump 9 min.; rest 1. Jump 9 min.	Jump 14 min.	Jump 4 min. Rest 1 min. (REPEAT × 3)	Rest.	Jump 1 min. Rest 1 min. (REPEAT × 12)	Jump 18 min.
5 EASY	Rest.	Jump 4 min.; rest 1. Jump 5 min.; rest 1. Jump 5 min.; rest 1. Jump 4 min.	Jump 9 min.	Jump 3 min. Rest 1 min. (REPEAT × 5)	Rest.	Jump 1 min. Rest 1 min. (REPEAT × 10)	Jump 16 min.
6 HARD	Rest.	Jump 10 min.; rest 1. Jump 6 min.; rest 1. Jump 4 min.	Jump 15 min.	Jump 5 min. Rest 1 min. (REPEAT × 4)	Rest.	Jump 1 min. Rest 1 min. (REPEAT × 15)	Jump 20 min.

JUMPING ROPE INTERMEDIATE   *6. Laying the Foundation*

JUMPING ROPE INTERMEDIATE 7. Building Endurance

DAY	1	Strength Work 2	3	Strength Work 4	5	Strength Work 6	7
WEEK 1 EASY	Rest.	Jump 5 min.; rest 1. Jump 9 min.; rest 1. Jump 4 min.; rest 1. Jump 3 min.	Jump 16 min.	Jump 7 min. Rest 1 min. (REPEAT × 3)	Rest.	Jump 1 min. Rest 1 min. (REPEAT × 14)	Jump 21 min.
2 MODERATE	Rest.	Jump 10 min., rest 1. Jump 8 min.; rest 1. Jump 5 min.	Jump 20 min.	Jump 6 min. Rest 1 min. (REPEAT × 4)	Rest.	Jump 1 min. Rest 1 min. (REPEAT × 18)	Jump 23 min.
3 EASY	Rest.	Jump 9 min.; rest 1. Jump 6 min.; rest 1. Jump 4 min.; rest 1. Jump 2 min.	Jump 9 min. Skip 6 min.	Jump 7 min. Rest 1 min. (REPEAT × 3)	Rest.	Jump 1 min. Rest 1 min. (REPEAT × 14)	Jump 22 min.
4 HARD	Rest.	Jump 12 min.; rest 1. Jump 12 min.	Jump 10 min. Skip 8 min.	Jump 7 min. Rest 1 min. (REPEAT × 4)	Rest.	Jump 2 min. Rest 1 min. (REPEAT × 12)	Jump 24 min.
5 EASY	Rest.	Jump 5 min.; rest 1. Jump 10 min.; rest 1. Jump 7 min.; rest 1. Jump 3 min.	Jump 10 min. Skip 10 min.	Jump 6 min. Rest 1 min. (REPEAT × 4)	Rest.	Jump 2 min. Rest 1 min. (REPEAT × 10)	Jump 25 min.
6 HARD	Rest.	Jump 16 min.; rest 1. Jump 10 min.	Rest.	Jump 8 min. Rest 1 min. (REPEAT × 4)	Rest.	Jump 2 min. Rest 1 min. (REPEAT × 13)	Jump 26 min.

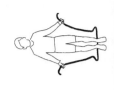

JUMPING ROPE INTERMEDIATE   *8. Achieving Mastery*

	DAY 1	Strength Work 2	3	Strength Work 4	5	Strength Work 6	7
WEEK 1 EASY	Rest.	Jump 8 min.; rest 1. Jump 6 min.; rest 1. Jump 5 min.; rest 1. Jump 3 min.	Jump 20 min. Skip 10 min.	Jump 5 min. Rest 1 min. (REPEAT × 5)	Rest.	Double jump 2 min. Rest 1 min. (REPEAT × 5)	Jump 25 min.
2 MODERATE	Rest.	Jump 8 min.; rest 1. Jump 12 min.; rest 1. Jump 8 min.	Jump 14 min. Skip 14 min.	Jump 5 min. Rest 1 min. (REPEAT × 6)	Rest.	Double jump 3 min. Rest 1 min. (REPEAT × 4)	Jump 28 min.
3 EASY	Rest.	Jump 8 min.; rest 1. Jump 7 min.; rest 1. Jump 6 min.; rest 1. Jump 4 min.	Rest.	Jump 4 min. Rest 1 min. (REPEAT × 6)	Rest.	Double jump 2 min. Rest 1 min. (REPEAT × 5)	Jump 26 min.
4 HARD	Rest.	Jump 20 min.; rest 1. Jump 5 min.	Jump 15 min. Skip 15 min.	Jump 3 min. Rest 1 min. (REPEAT × 6)	Rest.	Double jump 3 min. Rest 1 min. (REPEAT × 5)	Jump 30 min.
5 EASY							
6 HARD							

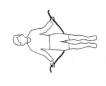

JUMPING ROPE ADVANCED   9. Awakening the Body

DAY	1	2 Strength Work	3	4 Strength Work	5	6 Strength Work	7
WEEK 1 EASY	Rest.	Jump 7 min.; rest 1. Jump 7 min.; rest 1. Jump 7 min.	Jump 8 min. Skip 10 min.	Double jump 5 min. Rest 1 min. (REPEAT × 5)	Rest.	Double jump 2 min. Rest 1 min. (REPEAT × 10)	Jump 31 min.
2 MODERATE	Rest.	Jump 10 min.; rest 1. Jump 10 min.; rest 1. Jump 10 min.	Rest.	Double jump 4 min. Rest 1 min. (REPEAT × 8)	Rest.	Double jump 2 min. Rest 1 min. (REPEAT × 12)	Jump 32 min.
3 EASY							
4 HARD							
5 EASY							
6 HARD							

DAY	1	Strength Work 2	3	Strength Work 4	5	Strength Work 6	7
WEEK 1 EASY	Rest.	Jump 10 min.; rest 1. Jump 7 min.; rest 1. Jump 7 min.; rest 1. Jump 10 min.	Jump 15 min. Skip 15 min.	Double jump 2 min. Rest 1 min. (REPEAT × 10)	Rest.	Double jump 2 min. Rest 1 min. (REPEAT × 11)	Jump 34 min.
2 MODERATE	Rest.	Jump 6 min.; rest 1. Jump 12 min.; rest 1. Jump 18 min.	Jump 16 min. Skip 16 min.	Double jump 3 min. Rest 1 min. (REPEAT × 12)	Rest.	Double jump 3 min. Rest 1 min. (REPEAT × 15)	Jump 36 min.
3 EASY	Rest.	Jump 12 min.; rest 1. Jump 9 min.; rest 1. Jump 8 min.; rest 1. Jump 7 min.	Rest.	Double jump 2 min. Rest 1 min. (REPEAT × 12)	Rest.	Double jump 3 min. Rest 1 min. (REPEAT × 10)	Jump 38 min.
4 HARD	Rest.	Jump 25 min.; rest 1. Jump 15 min.	Jump 20 min. Skip 20 min.	Double jump 4 min. Rest 1 min. (REPEAT × 10)	Rest.	Double jump 2 min. Rest 1 min. (REPEAT × 20)	Jump 40 min.
5 EASY	Rest.	Jump 18 min.; rest 1. Jump 14 min.; rest 1. Jump 10 min.; rest 1. Jump 8 min.	Game Day.	Double jump 3 min. Rest 1 min. (REPEAT × 10)	Rest.	Double jump 2 min. Rest 1 min. (REPEAT × 15)	Jump 41 min.
6 HARD	Rest.	Jump 17 min.; rest 1. Jump 25 min.	Game Day.	Double jump 5 min. Rest 1 min. (REPEAT × 5)	Rest.	Double jump 3 min. Rest 1 min. (REPEAT × 10)	Jump 42 min.

JUMPING ROPE ADVANCED   *10. Laying the Foundation*

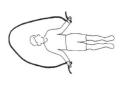

DAY / WEEK	1	2 Strength Work	3	4 Strength Work	5	6 Strength Work	7
1 EASY	Rest.	Jump 5 min.; rest 1. Jump 10 min.; rest 1. Jump 13 min.; rest 1. Jump 15 min.	Game Day.	Double jump 3 min. Rest 1 min. (REPEAT × 12)	Rest.	Double jump 2 min. Rest 1 min. (REPEAT × 15)	Jump 43 min.
2 MODERATE	Rest.	Jump 25 min.; rest 1. Jump 15 min.; rest 1. Jump 10 min.	Game Day.	Double jump 3 min. Rest 1 min. (REPEAT × 15)	Rest.	Double jump 4 min. Rest 1 min. (REPEAT × 15)	Jump 45 min.
3 EASY	Rest.	Jump 10 min.; rest 1. Jump 13 min.; rest 1. Jump 13 min.; rest 1. Jump 10 min.	Game Day.	Jump 25 min.	Rest.	Jump 30 min.	Jump 46 min.
4 HARD	Rest.	Jump 10 min. Skip 35 min.	Game Day.	Double jump 5 min. Rest 1 min. (REPEAT × 7)	Rest.	Double jump 5 min. Rest 1 min. (REPEAT × 8)	Jump 48 min.
5 EASY	Rest.	Jump 20 min.; rest 1. Jump 15 min.; rest 1. Jump 10 min.; rest 1. Jump 5 min.	Jump 25 min. Skip 25 min.	Game Day.	Rest.	Jump 40 min.	Jump 49 min.
6 HARD	Rest.	Jump 35 min. Skip 15 min.	Jump 15 min. Skip 35 min.	Game Day.	Rest.	Double jump 5 min. Rest 1 min. (REPEAT × 10)	Jump 52 min.

JUMPING ROPE ADVANCED   12. Achieving Mastery

DAY / WEEK	1	Strength Work 2	3	Strength Work 4	5	Strength Work 6	7
1 EASY	Rest.	Jump 15 min.; rest 1. Skip 10 min.; rest 1. Skip 10 min.; rest 1. Jump 15 min.	Jump 25 min.; rest 1. Skip 25 min.	Game Day.	Rest.	Jump 5 min. Skip 5 min. Rest 1 min. (REPEAT × 3)	Jump 54 min.
2 MODERATE	Rest.	Jump 15 min.; rest 1. Skip 16 min.; rest 1. Jump 30 min.	Jump 30 min.; rest 1. Skip 30 min.	Game Day.	Rest.	Double jump 5 min. Rest 1 min. (REPEAT × 10)	Jump 56 min.
3 EASY	Rest.	Jump 25 min.; rest 1. Skip 16 min.; rest 1. Skip 10 min.; rest 1. Jump 5 min.	Jump 30 min.; rest 1. Skip 30 min.	Game Day.	Rest.	Double jump 5 min. Rest 1 min. (REPEAT × 8)	Jump 58 min.
4 HARD	Rest.	Jump 30 min.; rest 1. Skip 30 min.	Jump 35 min.; rest 1. Skip 30 min.	Double jump 5 min. Rest 1 min. (REPEAT × 12)	Rest.	Double jump 5 min. Rest 1 min. (REPEAT × 10)	Jump 60 min.
5 EASY							
6 HARD							

DANCING

See art, pages 185–219.

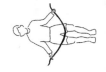

TECHNIQUE AND FORM

Because the disciplines of dance run the gamut from aerobics class at the local community college to professional ballet, tap, and jazz, no one formula can address all of its physical demands. But we do know one truth that spans that gamut. Human beings move to music naturally. Look down your row of seats next time you're at a concert and you will notice unconscious toe tapping, leg jiggling, finger thumping, and head bobbing all the way down the line. There is no question that we were all born to dance; it's just that some of us are better at it than others. Fortunately for those of us who are less skilled, some of those good dancers have found their ways into fitness centers and videotape studios, and adapted dance steps to provide rhythmic, systematic workouts for classes of willing students.

Before you begin the workout schedule, we assume that you already know how to dance. We don't assume that you're Broadway bound. You don't have to be in order to get a good workout. In getting aerobic benefit from dance, style doesn't count. Physical effort does. If you get your heart rate up, and have a good time, then you're succeeding. You can go aerobic or do mambo, samba, tap dance, waltz, or your own freestyle. The choice is entirely yours. It goes without saying that you are not going to be able to learn to dance from reading a book, including ours. If you need to be taught, we suggest that you study with a certified, experienced instructor. Ask to see credentials, interview the instructor before you sign up for the class, and talk to some other students. We want you to have fun, but we also want you to be safe and in competent, qualified hands!

EQUIPMENT YOU'LL NEED

A watch or clock

A bottle of water

Music—a CD or tape player, or a radio, or a dance workout videotape, a
    VCR, and a TV

WHAT TO WEAR

Wear clothing that is loose, cool, and comfortable. Everything's got to move with you. And it's got to wick sweat away from your body. Cotton is best.

Shoes: Purchase shoes that are specifically designed for dance. They are made to support and cushion the foot, but are flexible enough to move as you dance. (Note: don't wear running shoes. Their soles are designed to track your feet forward in the running gait, and impede any movement other than that.) When you shop for dance shoes, take along a pair of socks like the ones you intend to wear when you dance. Also, experts suggest that you try on the shoes at the same time of day you intend to work out, because the size of your foot may vary by as much as half a size during the course of your day. When you find a pair of shoes you like, try on *both* shoes. Lace them fully, and walk around the sales floor. Make sure you can get off the carpet and onto a firm surface if you really want to get a feel for how they'll perform for you in "real life"—unless you plan to dance only on carpet. Put the shoes through their paces. You don't need to perform the death scene from *Swan Lake,* but you do need to do a little fancy footwork. You need to road test these babies. (After you leave, the staff will talk about you only for a week or so . . . and then they'll forget.) Try on more than one pair and test each equally. Pay attention to raised surfaces, seams, and rough spots inside the shoe. Avoid being swayed by a shoe's appearance. It's what's inside and underneath that counts. In fact, we ask our clients to evaluate shoes with their eyes closed for at least a moment. In making your final decision about which shoes to buy, remember that comfort and fit are much more important than a fancy sales pitch from a clerk who may or may not be particularly knowledgeable about shoes and the biomechanics of dancing. *You* take charge here. After all, you're going to be working out in the shoes.

Socks: Socks are optional, but most dancers appreciate them. They add a layer of protection between your foot and the inside of the shoe. Look for a smooth, snug fit that's free from wrinkles and inside seams. Because even the best socks are an inexpensive investment, go first-class. Purchase athletes' socks that are engineered to wick moisture, or absorb sweat away from your foot and provide you with a dryer shoe interior, which will help prevent blistering, skin irritations, and odor. Treat yourself to a clean pair of socks with every workout.

BOREDOM BUSTERS

Recruit a partner: Dancing is always more fun if you share it with a friend. You and a friend can work together to keep your training schedules on track. Better yet, join a club or a dance group.

Go out dancing: If you enjoy dancing, take the one you love and do it on a real dance floor. Make an evening of it.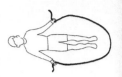

Vary your music, vary your style: No need to get stuck in a rut when there is so much music in the world and so many styles of dance. If you need fresh rhythms, but don't want to spend any money, go to the library and borrow a new CD or tape, or download music from the Internet (legally, please).

Participate in an event: Find a dance-a-thon and join in the fun. Just be sure you can handle the physical demands of the event so that your performance doesn't turn into a personal version of *They Shoot Horses, Don't They?*

Attend an event: Dance is performance art. Lucky for you, artists tour the country constantly. If you're a big fan of ballet and an aspiring ballet dancer, get thee to the theater and revel in the wonderfulness of your chosen dance. One evening of seeing how it's really done will inspire you for months.

TAKING IT TO THE GYM
Dance classes

INJURY ALERT

In recent years, a large percentage of our practice has been treating injured professional dancers. Surprised? Don't be. Certainly professional dancers are athletic—strong and flexible. But dancers are sometimes more concerned with form (how they look) and less concerned with function (how they got into position). And this lack of understanding puts them at risk. To compound the problem, dancers force their bodies into extreme attitudes that can easily exceed human physical limitations . . . and they insist on making it all look easy. Injuries are usually the result of creeping, chronic mistakes that sneak up on dancers and knock the legs right out from under them when they can least afford downtime.

The most common injuries in dancers are in the lumbar spine, and are the results of arching—flexing and extending the back—with improper alignment and imbalances in the tendons and muscles. Experts agree that strong abdominals, and lengthened hip flexors and thoracolumbar fascia, are essential before submitting the spine to the demands of dance without injury. And, of course, proper warm-up is critical.

In recreational dancers, we see a lot of tender feet, knees, and hips from dancing on a surface that's a little too hard and wearing shoes that are a little too soft. Avoid these problems with proper warm-up and by making sure you're absorbing impact properly.

TIPS FROM THE EXPERTS

You need to supplement your dance program with strength training—particularly for upper body—and flexibility work to offset the pounding your lower body takes in dance. Pay attention to your body. Buy the best shoes you can afford. When injury strikes, seek advice from a physician who treats athletes and their injuries. And, once you get that advice, heed it. Be smart and you'll live to dance another day.

Please remember to hydrate. Even slight dehydration lowers the circulating volume of blood and causes the core temperature to rise. The more dehydrated the dancer becomes, the more dangerous the situation gets. Symptoms of progressive dehydration include fatigue, lack of coordination, muscle pain and cramping, headache, light-headedness, confusion, disorientation, and fainting. Under extreme circumstances, death can occur. If you feel thirsty, you're already on your way to trouble. Drink early—before thirst sets in—and often. Experts say that water is perfect for short events, but a commercial sport fluid-replacement drink is preferable for events of more than ninety minutes in duration. With either choice, *cold* is best. We want you to play it cool, twinkle toes. Drink.

COMING TO TERMS WITH THE TERMS WE USE IN YOUR SCHEDULE

Easy effort: This is a leisurely, conversational pace. You should be in the minimum range of your target heart rate.

Moderate effort: This is a quickened pace, but still conversational. You should be in the middle range of your target heart rate.

Hard effort: Now you're working. At this point, conversation might be difficult. You should be in the higher ranges of your target heart rate.

DANCING BEGINNER · *1. Awakening the Body*

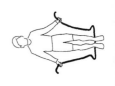

DAY	1	Strength Work 2	3	Strength Work 4	5	Strength Work 6	7
WEEK 1 EASY	Make sure your music, shoes, and clothing are in order.	Dance 15 min. Easy effort.	Dance 15 min. Easy effort.	Dance 15 min. Moderate effort.	Rest.	Dance 5 min. Easy effort. Dance 15 min. Moderate effort.	Dance 5 min. Easy effort. Dance 15 min. Moderate effort.
2 MODERATE	Rest.	Dance 5 min. Easy effort. Dance 15 min. Moderate effort Dance 5 min. Easy effort.	Dance 15 min. Easy effort.	Rest.	Dance 5 min. Easy effort. Dance 15 min. Moderate effort. Dance 5 min. Easy effort.	Rest.	Dance 5 min. Easy effort. Dance 15 min. Moderate effort.
3 EASY							
4 HARD							
5 EASY							
6 HARD							

DANCING BEGINNER *2. Laying the Foundation*

DAY / WEEK	1	Strength Work 2	3	Strength Work 4	5	Strength Work 6	7
1 EASY	Rest.	Dance 20 min. Easy effort.	Dance 10 min. Easy effort. Dance 15 min. Moderate effort. Dance 10 min. Easy effort.	Dance 20 min. Easy effort.	Rest.	Dance 20 min. Easy effort.	Dance 5 min. Easy effort. Dance 20 min. Moderate effort.
2 MODERATE	Rest.	Dance 10 min. Easy effort. Dance 20 min. Moderate effort. Dance 10 min. Easy effort.	Dance 20 min. Easy effort.	Rest.	Dance 5 min. Easy effort. Dance 20 min. Moderate effort. Dance 5 min. Easy effort.	Rest.	Dance 10 min. Easy effort. Dance 5 min. Moderate effort. Dance 10 min. Easy effort.
3 EASY	Rest.	Dance 25 min. Easy effort.	Rest.	Dance 20 min. Easy effort.	Rest.	Dance 5 min. Easy effort. Dance 20 min. Moderate effort.	Dance 5 min. Easy effort. Dance 20 min. Moderate effort. Dance 5 min. Easy effort.
4 HARD	Rest.	Dance 5 min. Easy effort. Dance 20 min. Moderate effort. Dance 5 min. Easy effort.	Dance 25 min. Moderate effort. Dance 5 min. Easy effort.	Dance 5 min. Easy effort. Dance 5 min. Moderate effort. Dance 5 min. Easy effort.	Rest.	Dance 20 min. Easy effort.	Dance 20 min. Easy effort.
5 EASY	Rest.	Dance 5 min. Easy effort. Dance 20 min. Moderate effort. Dance 5 min. Easy effort.	Rest.	Rest.	Dance 5 min. Easy effort. Dance 20 min. Moderate effort. Dance 5 min. Easy effort.	Rest.	Dance 5 min. Easy effort. Dance 10 min. Moderate effort. Dance 10 min. Easy effort.
6 HARD	Rest.	Dance 30 min. Easy effort.	Dance 5 min. Easy effort. Dance 20 min. Moderate effort. Dance 5 min. Easy effort.	Dance 10 min. Easy effort. Dance 5 min. Moderate effort. Dance 10 min. Easy effort.	Rest.	Dance 20 min. Easy effort.	Dance 5 min. Easy effort. Dance 10 min. Moderate effort. Dance 10 min. Easy effort.

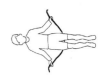

DAY	1	2 Strength Work	3	4 Strength Work	5	6 Strength Work	7
WEEK 1 EASY	Rest.	Dance 5 min. Easy effort. Dance 10 min. Moderate effort. Dance 10 min. Easy effort.	Dance 5 min. Easy effort. Dance 10 min. Moderate effort. Dance 5 min. Easy effort.	Rest.	Dance 5 min. Easy effort. Dance 15 min. Moderate effort. Dance 5 min. Easy effort.	Rest.	Dance 5 min. Easy effort. Dance 15 min. Moderate effort. Dance 5 min. Easy effort.
2 MODERATE	Rest.	Dance 5 min. Easy effort. Dance 15 min. Moderate effort. Dance 10 min. Easy effort.	Dance 5 min. Easy effort. Dance 10 min. Moderate effort. Dance 5 min. Easy effort.	Dance 10 min. Easy effort. Dance 15 min. Moderate effort. Dance 5 min. Easy effort.	Rest.	Dance 5 min. Easy effort. Dance 15 min. Moderate effort. Dance 10 min. Easy effort.	Dance 5 min. Easy effort. Dance 20 min. Moderate effort. Dance 5 min. Easy effort.
3 EASY	Rest.	Dance 5 min. Easy effort. Dance 10 min. Moderate effort. Dance 10 min. Easy effort.	Dance 5 min. Easy effort. Dance 10 min. Moderate effort. Dance 5 min. Easy effort.	Rest.	Dance 5 min. Easy effort. Dance 15 min. Moderate effort. Dance 10 min. Easy effort.	Rest.	Dance 5 min. Easy effort. Dance 15 min. Moderate effort. Dance 5 min. Easy effort.
4 HARD	Rest.	Dance 5 min. Easy effort. Dance 20 min. Moderate effort. Dance 5 min. Easy effort.	Dance 5 min. Easy effort. Dance 15 min. Moderate effort. Dance 5 min. Easy effort.	Dance 10 min. Easy effort. Dance 20 min. Moderate effort. Dance 5 min. Easy effort.	Rest.	Dance 5 min. Easy effort. Dance 20 min. Moderate effort. Dance 5 min. Easy effort.	Dance 15 min. Easy effort. Dance 20 min. Moderate effort. Dance 5 min. Easy effort.
5 EASY	Rest.	Dance 5 min. Easy effort. Dance 15 min. Moderate effort. Dance 10 min. Easy effort.	Dance 5 min. Easy effort. Dance 20 min. Moderate effort. Dance 5 min. Easy effort.	Rest.	Dance 5 min. Easy effort. Dance 10 min. Moderate effort. Dance 5 min. Easy effort.	Rest.	Dance 25 min. Moderate effort.
6 HARD	Rest.	Dance 5 min. Easy effort. Dance 10 min. Moderate effort. Dance 15 min. Easy effort.	Dance 5 min. Easy effort. Dance 25 min. Moderate effort. Dance 5 min. Easy effort.	Dance 10 min. Easy effort. Dance 20 min. Moderate effort. Dance 5 min. Easy effort.	Rest.	Dance 5 min. Easy effort. Dance 10 min. Moderate effort. Dance 5 min. Easy effort.	Dance 30 min. Moderate effort

DANCING BEGINNER 4. *Achieving Mastery*

DAY	1	2 Strength Work	3	4 Strength Work	5	6 Strength Work	7
WEEK 1 EASY	Rest.	Dance 5 min. Easy effort. Dance 25 min. Moderate effort. Dance 5 min. Easy effort.	Dance 5 min. Easy effort. Dance 15 min. Moderate effort. Dance 5 min. Easy effort.	Rest.	Dance 10 min. Easy effort. Dance 15 min. Moderate effort. Dance 5 min. Easy effort.	Dance 5 min. Easy effort. Dance 20 min. Moderate effort. Dance 5 min. Easy effort.	Dance 5 min. Easy effort. Dance 25 min. Moderate effort. Dance 5 min. Easy effort.
2 MODERATE	Rest.	Dance 5 min. Easy effort. Dance 25 min. Moderate effort. Dance 5 min. Easy effort.	Dance 5 min. Easy effort. Dance 20 min. Moderate effort. Dance 5 min. Easy effort.	Dance 5 min. Easy effort. Dance 15 min. Moderate effort. Dance 5 min. Easy effort.	Rest.	Dance 5 min. Easy effort. Dance 10 min. Moderate effort. Dance 5 min. Easy effort.	Dance 20 min. Easy effort. Dance 10 min. Moderate effort. Dance 5 min. Easy effort.
3 EASY							
4 HARD							
5 EASY							
6 HARD							

DANCING INTERMEDIATE   5. Awakening the Body

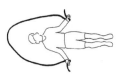

DAY	1	Strength Work 2	3	Strength Work 4	5	Strength Work 6	7
WEEK 1 EASY	Rest.	Dance 5 min. Easy effort. Dance 25 min. Moderate effort. Dance 5 min. Easy effort.	Dance 5 min. Easy effort. Dance 15 min. Moderate effort. Dance 5 min. Easy effort.	Dance 5 min. Easy effort. Dance 20 min. Moderate effort. Dance 5 min. Easy effort.	Rest.	Dance 10 min. Easy effort. Dance 15 min. Moderate effort. Dance 5 min. Easy effort.	Dance 20 min. Easy effort. Dance 10 min. Moderate effort. Dance 10 min. Easy effort.
2 MODERATE	Rest.	Dance 5 min. Easy effort. Dance 25 min. Moderate effort. Dance 5 min. Easy effort.	Dance 5 min. Easy effort. Dance 20 min. Moderate effort. Dance 5 min. Easy effort.	Dance 5 min. Easy effort. Dance 25 min. Moderate effort. Dance 5 min. Easy effort.	Rest.	Dance 10 min. Easy effort. Dance 20 min. Moderate effort. Dance 5 min. Easy effort.	Dance 10 min. Easy effort. Dance 20 min. Moderate effort. Dance 5 min. Easy effort.
3 EASY							
4 HARD							
5 EASY							
6 HARD							

DAY	1	Strength Work			5	Strength Work	
	1	2	3	4	5	6	7
WEEK 1 EASY	Rest.	Dance 20 min. Easy effort.	Dance 5 min. Easy effort. Dance 15 min. Moderate effort. Dance 5 min. Easy effort.	Dance 10 min. Easy effort. Dance 25 min. Moderate effort. Dance 5 min. Easy effort.	Rest.	Dance 10 min. Easy effort. Dance 20 min. Moderate effort. Dance 5 min. Easy effort.	Dance 10 min. Easy effort. Dance 20 min. Moderate effort. Dance 5 min. Easy effort.
WEEK 2 MODERATE	Rest.	Dance 20 min. Easy effort. Dance 10 min. Moderate effort. Dance 5 min. Easy effort.	Dance 5 min. Easy effort. Dance 20 min. Moderate effort. Dance 5 min. Easy effort.	Dance 5 min. Easy effort. Dance 35 min. Moderate effort. Dance 5 min. Easy effort.	Rest.	Dance 5 min. Easy effort. Dance 25 min. Moderate effort. Dance 5 min. Easy effort.	Dance 10 min. Easy effort. Dance 20 min. Moderate effort. Dance 5 min. Easy effort.
WEEK 3 EASY	Rest.	Dance 20 min. Easy effort. Dance 10 min. Hard effort. Dance 5 min. Moderate effort.	Dance 15 min. Easy effort. Dance 10 min. Hard effort. Dance 5 min. Moderate effort.	Dance 5 min. Easy effort. Dance 10 min. Hard effort. Dance 15 min. Moderate effort.	Rest.	Dance 35 min. Moderate effort.	Dance 10 min. Easy effort. Dance 20 min. Moderate effort. Dance 5 min. Easy effort.
WEEK 4 HARD	Rest.	Dance 20 min. Moderate effort. Dance 10 min. Hard effort. Dance 5 min. Moderate effort.	Dance 5 min. Moderate effort. Dance 20 min. Hard effort. Dance 5 min. Moderate effort.	Dance 5 min. Moderate effort. Dance 5 min. Hard effort. Dance 5 min. Moderate effort. Repeat set twice.	Rest.	Dance 25 min. Easy effort. Dance 5 min. Moderate effort. Dance 5 min. Easy effort.	Dance 10 min. Easy effort. Dance 20 min. Moderate effort. Dance 5 min. Easy effort.
WEEK 5 EASY	Rest.	Dance 10 min. Moderate effort. Dance 5 min. Hard effort. Dance 5 min. Moderate effort.	Dance 10 min. Moderate effort. Dance 10 min. Hard effort. Dance 5 min. Moderate effort.	Dance 20 min. Moderate effort. Dance 10 min. Hard effort. Dance 5 min. Moderate effort.	Rest.	Dance 5 min. Easy effort. Dance 20 min. Moderate effort. Dance 5 min. Easy effort.	Dance 10 min. Easy effort. Dance 20 min. Moderate effort. Dance 5 min. Easy effort.
WEEK 6 HARD	Rest.	Dance 10 min. Moderate effort. Dance 20 min. Hard effort. Dance 5 min. Moderate effort.	Dance 10 min. Moderate effort. Dance 25 min. Hard effort. Dance 5 min. Moderate effort.	Dance 5 min. Moderate effort. Dance 35 min. Hard effort. Dance 5 min. Moderate effort.	Rest.	Dance 10 min. Easy effort. Dance 10 min. Moderate effort. Dance 5 min. Hard effort.	Dance 10 min. Easy effort. Dance 20 min. Moderate effort. Dance 5 min. Easy effort.

DANCING INTERMEDIATE   *6. Laying the Foundation*

DAY	1	Strength Work 2	3	Strength Work 4	5	Strength Work 6	7
WEEK 1 EASY	Rest.	Dance 15 min. Moderate effort. Dance 5 min. Hard effort.	Dance 5 min. Moderate effort. Dance 5 min. Hard effort. Dance 5 min. Moderate effort.	Dance 5 min. Moderate effort. Dance 10 min. Hard effort. Dance 5 min. Moderate effort.	Rest.	Dance 20 min. Moderate effort. Dance 5 min. Hard effort. Dance 5 min. Moderate effort.	Dance 30 min. Moderate effort.
2 MODERATE	Rest.	Dance 20 min. Moderate effort. Dance 10 min. Hard effort.	Dance 10 min. Moderate effort. Dance 5 min. Hard effort. Dance 5 min. Moderate effort.	Dance 5 min. Moderate effort. Dance 15 min. Hard effort. Dance 5 min. Moderate effort.	Rest.	Dance 15 min. Moderate effort. Dance 10 min. Hard effort. Dance 5 min. Moderate effort.	Dance 20 min. Hard effort.
3 EASY	Rest.	Dance 15 min. Moderate effort. Dance 5 min. Hard effort.	Dance 15 min. Moderate effort. Dance 10 min. Hard effort. Dance 5 min. Moderate effort.	Dance 5 min. Moderate effort. Dance 10 min. Hard effort. Dance 5 min. Moderate effort.	Rest.	Dance 20 min. Moderate effort. Dance 5 min. Hard effort. Dance 5 min. Moderate effort.	Dance 20 min. Hard effort.
4 HARD	Rest.	Dance 20 min. Moderate effort. Dance 5 min. Hard effort.	Dance 15 min. Moderate effort. Dance 10 min. Hard effort. Dance 5 min. Moderate effort.	Dance 5 min. Moderate effort. Dance 10 min. Hard effort. Dance 5 min. Moderate effort.	Rest.	Dance 15 min. Moderate effort. Dance 15 min. Hard effort. Dance 5 min. Moderate effort.	Dance 30 min. Moderate effort.
5 EASY	Rest.	Dance 20 min. Moderate effort. Dance 5 min. Hard effort.	Dance 15 min. Moderate effort. Dance 10 min. Hard effort. Dance 5 min. Moderate effort.	Dance 5 min. Moderate effort. Dance 10 min. Hard effort. Dance 5 min. Moderate effort.	Rest.	Dance 15 min. Easy effort. Dance 10 min. Moderate effort. Dance 5 min. Hard effort.	Dance 20 min. Hard effort.
6 HARD	Rest.	Dance 25 min. Moderate effort. Dance 5 min. Hard effort.	Rest.	Dance 10 min. Moderate effort. Dance 10 min. Hard effort. Dance 5 min. Moderate effort.	Rest.	Dance 30 min. Moderate effort.	Dance 20 min. Hard effort.

DANCING INTERMEDIATE *7. Building Endurance*

DANCING INTERMEDIATE   *8. Achieving Mastery*

DAY	1	Strength Work — 2	3	Strength Work — 4	5	Strength Work — 6	7
WEEK 1 EASY	Rest.	Dance 35 min. Hard effort.	Dance 5 min. Moderate effort. Dance 10 min. Hard effort. Dance 5 min. Moderate effort.	Dance 10 min. Moderate effort. Dance 10 min. Hard effort. Dance 10 min. Moderate effort.	Rest.	Dance 15 min. Moderate effort. Dance 10 min. Hard effort.	Dance 35 min. Hard effort. Dance 5 min. Moderate effort.
2 MODERATE	Rest.	Dance 35 min. Hard effort.	Dance 5 min. Moderate effort. Dance 15 min. Hard effort. Dance 5 min. Moderate effort.	Dance 25 min. Hard effort. Dance 5 min. Moderate effort.	Rest.	Dance 20 min. Moderate effort. Dance 15 min. Hard effort. Dance 5 min. Moderate effort.	Dance 35 min. Hard effort. Dance 5 min. Moderate effort.
3 EASY	Rest.	Dance 35 min. Hard effort.	Rest.	Dance 25 min. Hard effort. Dance 5 min. Moderate effort.	Rest.	Dance 10 min. Moderate effort. Dance 10 min. Hard effort. Dance 5 min. Moderate effort.	Dance 35 min. Hard effort. Dance 5 min. Moderate effort.
4 HARD	Rest.	Dance 35 min. Hard effort.	Dance 20 min. Hard effort. Dance 5 min. Moderate effort.	Dance 25 min. Hard effort. Dance 5 min. Moderate effort.	Rest.	Dance 10 min. Moderate effort. Dance 15 min. Hard effort. Dance 5 min. Moderate effort.	Dance 35 min. Hard effort. Dance 5 min. Moderate effort.
5 EASY							
6 HARD							

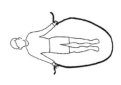

DANCING ADVANCED *9. Awakening the Body*

DAY	1	Strength Work 2	3	Strength Work 4	5	Strength Work 6	7
WEEK 1 EASY	Rest.	Dance 25 min. Hard effort. Dance 5 min. Moderate effort.	Dance 35 min. Hard effort.	Dance 5 min. Moderate effort. Dance 15 min. Hard effort. Dance 5 min. Moderate effort.	Rest.	Dance 20 min. Moderate effort. Dance 10 min. Hard effort. Dance 5 min. Moderate effort.	Dance 40 min. Hard effort. Dance 5 min. Moderate effort.
2 MODERATE	Rest.	Dance 30 min. Hard effort. Dance 5 min. Moderate effort.	Rest.	Dance 25 min. Hard effort. Dance 5 min. Moderate effort.	Rest.	Dance 40 min. Moderate effort.	Dance 45 min. Hard effort. Dance 5 min. Moderate effort.
3 EASY							
4 HARD							
5 EASY							
6 HARD							

DAY	1	Strength Work 2	3	Strength Work 4	5	Strength Work 6	7
WEEK 1 EASY	Rest.	Dance 35 min. Hard effort. Dance 5 min. Moderate effort.	Dance 5 min. Moderate effort. Dance 35 min. Hard effort. Dance 5 min. Moderate effort.	Dance 15 min. Moderate effort. Dance 10 min. Hard effort. Dance 5 min. Moderate effort.	Rest.	Dance 20 min. Moderate effort. Dance 10 min. Hard effort.	Dance 30 min. Moderate effort. Dance 5 min. Hard effort.
2 MODERATE	Rest.	Dance 35 min. Hard effort. Dance 5 min. Moderate effort.	Dance 5 min. Moderate effort. Dance 40 min. Hard effort. Dance 5 min. Moderate effort.	Dance 20 min. Moderate effort. Dance 10 min. Hard effort. Dance 5 min. Moderate effort.	Rest.	Dance 20 min. Moderate effort.	Dance 40 min. Moderate effort. Dance 5 min. Hard effort.
3 EASY	Rest.	Dance 35 min. Hard effort. Dance 5 min. Moderate effort.	Rest.	Dance 10 min. Moderate effort. Dance 10 min. Hard effort. Dance 5 min. Moderate effort.	Rest.	Dance 10 min. Moderate effort. Dance 30 min. Hard effort.	Dance 40 min. Moderate effort. Dance 5 min. Hard effort.
4 HARD	Rest.	Dance 35 min. Hard effort. Dance 5 min. Moderate effort.	Dance 5 min. Moderate effort. Dance 40 min. Hard effort. Dance 5 min. Moderate effort.	Dance 25 min. Moderate effort. Dance 15 min. Hard effort. Dance 5 min. Moderate effort.	Rest.	Dance 20 min. Moderate effort. Dance 5 min. Hard effort.	Dance 35 min. Moderate effort. Dance 10 min. Hard effort.
5 EASY	Rest.	Dance 35 min. Hard effort. Dance 5 min. Moderate effort.	Game Day.	Dance 20 min. Moderate effort. Dance 10 min. Hard effort.	Rest.	Dance 20 min. Moderate effort. Dance 20 min. Hard effort.	Dance 30 min. Moderate effort. Dance 10 min. Hard effort.
6 HARD	Rest.	Dance 35 min. Hard effort. Dance 5 min. Moderate effort.	Game Day.	Dance 15 min. Moderate effort. Dance 30 min. Hard effort.	Rest.	Dance 20 min. Moderate effort. Dance 10 min. Hard effort.	Dance 40 min. Moderate effort. Dance 10 min. Hard effort.

DANCING ADVANCED   *10. Laying the Foundation*

DAY	1	Strength Work 2	3	Strength Work 4	5	Strength Work 6	7
WEEK 1 EASY	Rest.	Dance 30 min. Hard effort.	Game Day.	Dance 10 min. Moderate effort. Dance 20 min. Hard effort. Dance 5 min. Moderate effort.	Rest.	Dance 10 min. Moderate effort. Dance 20 min. Hard effort.	Dance 30 min. Hard effort.
2 MODERATE	Rest.	Dance 40 min. Hard effort.	Game Day.	Dance 10 min. Moderate effort. Dance 30 min. Hard effort. Dance 5 min. Moderate effort.	Rest.	Dance 20 min. Moderate effort. Dance 20 min. Hard effort.	Dance 40 min. Hard effort.
3 EASY	Rest.	Dance 30 min. Hard effort.	Game Day.	Dance 45 min. Hard effort.	Rest.	Dance 20 min. Moderate effort. Dance 20 min. Hard effort.	Dance 45 min. Moderate effort.
4 HARD	Rest.	Dance 45 min. Hard effort.	Game Day.	Dance 45 min. Hard effort.	Rest.	Dance 20 min. Moderate effort. Dance 20 min. Hard effort.	Dance 50 min. Hard effort.
5 EASY	Rest.	Dance 10 min. Moderate effort. Dance 20 min. Hard effort. Dance 5 min. Moderate effort.	Dance 40 min. Hard effort.	Game Day.	Rest.	Dance 30 min. Hard effort.	Dance 45 min. Hard effort.
6 HARD	Rest.	Dance 10 min. Moderate effort. Dance 20 min. Hard effort. Dance 10 min. Moderate effort.	Dance 45 min. Hard effort.	Game Day.	Rest.	Dance 30 min. Hard effort.	Dance 50 min. Hard effort.

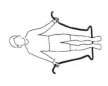

DANCING ADVANCED *11. Building Endurance*

DAY	1	Strength Work 2	3	Strength Work 4	5	Strength Work 6	7
WEEK 1 EASY	Rest.	Dance 10 min. Moderate effort. Dance 20 min. Hard effort. Dance 5 min. Moderate effort.	Dance 50 min. Hard effort.	Game Day.	Rest.	Dance 30 min. Hard effort.	Dance 45 min. Hard effort.
2 MODERATE	Rest.	Dance 10 min. Moderate effort. Dance 30 min. Hard effort. Dance 5 min. Moderate effort.	Dance 50 min. Hard effort.	Game Day.	Rest.	Dance 30 min. Hard effort.	Dance 55 min. Hard effort.
3 EASY	Rest.	Dance 5 min. Moderate effort. Dance 35 min. Hard effort. Dance 10 min. Moderate effort.	Dance 30 min. Hard effort.	Game Day.	Rest.	Dance 30 min. Hard effort.	Dance 45 min. Hard effort.
4 HARD	Rest.	Dance 35 min. Hard effort.	Dance 40 min. Hard effort.	Dance 30 min. Hard effort.	Rest.	Dance 40 min. Hard effort.	Dance 60 min. Hard effort.
5 EASY							
6 HARD							

DANCING ADVANCED   *12. Achieving Mastery*

SWIMMING

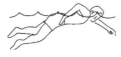 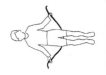

See art, pages 221–237.

TECHNIQUE AND FORM

We assume that you already know how to swim before beginning this swimming program, and are familiar with a few basic strokes. If not, your experience in the pool is going to be a short, unpleasant one that will probably involve a cranky lifeguard. It goes without saying that swimming can't be learned from a book, and it certainly can't be learned from this small section. If you can't swim, sign up for lessons with the best coach you can find, or register for a class taught by the Red Cross or the local YMCA. This program will be useful after you've developed some skills and proficiencies.

As trainers, we like swimming. We often use it to keep endurance athletes fit while we rehabilitate injuries, because it provides a remarkable cardiovascular and muscular workout without pounding the joints. The support of the water takes all the weight off fragile body parts. This is why we also highly recommend swimming for formerly inactive beginning athletes who might not be well suited to hard charging . . . yet. But this positive aspect of swimming is also a negative. Swimming is not load-bearing, meaning that it doesn't give the bones the benefit of mild stress and gravity (such as would be found in walking or running). Bones are living, dynamic tissues that regenerate and remodel themselves constantly. Those that are mildly stressed—loaded—rebuild more strongly and quickly than bones that aren't. The ability to help build skeletal integrity with exercise has significant consequences, especially later in life. For example, osteoporosis, the loss of calcium in bone, can be slowed, and slightly reversed, with load-bearing activity. Because swimming isn't load-bearing, you will find it necessary to engage in some dry-land activities like walking.

Although there are many ways to swim, there are four basic strokes in competitive swimming: the crawl, the backstroke, the breaststroke, and the butterfly. The strokes have four common aspects—reach out, catch the water, pull the body using the resistance of the water, and recover by returning the body to neutral before beginning the cycle again. Each stroke has its individual biomechanics, but they all have one thing in common: they add to a superior workout.

Olympic silver medalist Allison Wagner, who helped us develop this workout schedule, recommends that you begin your program by locating a shortcourse pool—one that is twenty-five yards or twenty-five meters from deck to deck. Beware the fifty-meter pool! Allison warns that for a beginner, bigger is not better, at least not at first. A short-course pool is long enough and might even be longer than you think. When you enter the pool for the first time, you might not be sure how much stamina you have. Swim your first lap close to the side and make sure you have energy enough to get from one end to the other before you venture out into the middle. If you're close to the side and poop out, you can merely reach over and hang on until you get your second wind. Try to start your lap from the shallow end of the pool. (Most recreational pools have a shallow end that slopes down to a deep end.) If you can't complete the lap, you'll still be in water you can stand in, or not too far beyond that point. Turn around and head back.

Each workout will begin with a training technique that makes Allison the champion she is: bobbing to enhance breath control.

EQUIPMENT YOU'LL NEED

Watch (waterproof!)
Bottle of water
Towel
Kickboard
Pull buoy

WHAT TO WEAR

Bathing suit, goggles and a cap (optional). Make sure the suit you choose is one that is designed for swimming, as opposed to one that looks good. You'll want a tight fit to reduce drag as you move through the water, and you might want one that dries quickly . . . like immediately.

For women only: Make sure the straps on your suit are comfortable and won't cut into your shoulders or slide off as you rotate your arms. Also, make sure there is little or no gap between the suit and your skin at the breast. If there is, as you move though the water, that little gap will fill with water, causing resistance that will either pull your suit down or create drag to slow you. If you're fighting to keep your suit up, you're not able to enjoy the full benefit of your swim.

BOREDOM BUSTERS

Listen to music: A waterproof CD or tape player, or radio with lightweight headset might be fun for a while. Just make sure that your choice of music is compatible with your planned workout. You'll want a steady tempo. (This is

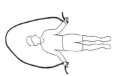

for beginners only. As your workouts increase in intensity, you won't be able to keep a headset on as you torpedo through the water.)

Recruit a partner: While it's true that conversation is impossible when you're facedown in the pool, it's fun to work out with a friend in the next lane. A little support and friendly competition go a long way in improving performance levels. Also, you'll keep each other on schedule.

Join a club: There are clubs and classes in almost every community where you can meet other swimmers and coaches to share the fun and keep your training fresh and exciting. Other swimmers are wonderful sources of information regarding technique, equipment, and competitive events.

Sign up to compete in a swim meet: There's nothing that puts more focus and sparkle into your training than a goal: a specific event on a specific date. No matter what level you're on, you'll be a welcome addition to the competition . . . and you might even swim away with a medal!

Be present: One of the skills most of us have lost in our hectic lives is the ability to just *be.* We're always reviewing things that have already happened or planning what's about to happen. Being in the moment is a particular challenge made more easy by the solitude the water imposes on you. You can't hear anything anyway, so why not just be?

Pennies: If you're swimming laps, line up pennies on the deck at the far end of the pool: one for each lap. Swim to the pennies and take one. Return it to the end of the pool at which you began the lap. Put it on the deck. Swim to the other pennies and take one more. Return it to the end of the pool at which you began the lap. Repeat this until all the pennies have been moved from the far end of the pool to the near end.

Play: Being weightless and buoyant in the water is wonderful. Take a few minutes to do handstands, somersaults, and gravity-defying acrobatics, and enjoy yourself. That's what swimming is for.

TAKING IT TO THE GYM
Indoor pool

INJURY ALERT
Shoulder injuries account for most of the injuries endemic to swimming. Little wonder. It's the most mobile joint in the body, yet it has little skeletal support, relying instead on the shoulder capsule, the rotator cuff, tendons, ligaments, and muscles in the upper arm, shoulder, and upper back. The relationship is

elegant, but it breaks down now and then. Overuse injuries head the list with contributions from poor form in the water, overtraining, poor training techniques, fatigue, inflexibility, compromised blood supply to the shoulder, weakness, skeletal anomalies, untreated irritations and inflammations, imbalance, instability in the joint, and impingements caused by stroking. The possibilities seem endless and daunting, yet a little intelligence goes a long way in preventing injury.

Injuries can be largely prevented with training that swimmers call dry-land training: strength, flexibility, and cardiovascular work. Second, work with a coach to be certain that your technique is perfect. Nothing will slow you down more or guarantee an injury faster than poor technique. And third, remember that overuse injuries can often be avoided by conditioning—working up to manage the demand slowly. Be careful to *gradually* increase your time in the water. Fatigue is an important contributor to injury. If you're not physically ready to do the work, and wear yourself out trying, you're headed toward injury. And finally, pay close attention to minor aches and pains, especially in the shoulders. Research demonstrates conclusively that shoulder problems start small. You may be able to head off a larger problem by dealing with a minor irritation.

TIPS FROM THE EXPERTS

Although swimming is a wonderful exercise, it isn't a load-bearing exercise—that is, swimming doesn't put any impact on the bones. Women who rely on exercise for osteoporosis prevention need load-bearing work and should consider adding some more appropriate fitness components to their training, such as walking or running.

Finally, never let it be said, "Water, water everywhere and not a drop to drink!" Remember to put your full water bottle within easy reach and stay hydrated when you swim. It's easy to forget that you're working hard, heating up, and sweating while you're in cool water. But failing to maintain your fluids will cause you to fatigue and lose function.

COMING TO TERMS WITH THE TERMS WE USE IN YOUR SCHEDULE

Easy effort: This is a leisurely pace. You should be in the minimum range of your target heart rate.

Moderate effort: This is a quickened pace, but still relaxed. You should be in the middle range of your target heart rate.

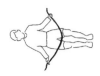

Hard effort: This is race pace. You should be in the higher ranges of your target heart rate.

Time and distance: Of course, the logical way to organize a swimming schedule would be to specify laps, but pools come in all shapes and sizes, so you'll have to determine how many laps are equal to the times we're suggesting. It's not necessary to be precise, as long as you're close.

Bob: This is Olympic silver medalist Allison Wagner's secret for enhancing her ability to breathe and, equally important, hold her breath while she's swimming. Pick an area of the pool where you can stand with your feet on the bottom and your head out of the water. Take a deep breath and submerge your head and let out *all* the air in your lungs. Hold still for a moment, then return to the surface to take another breath. Recover. When you're ready, exhale and submerge again.

Strokes: Notice we don't specify strokes. Although they are important to being a swimmer, they are not particularly important to working out cardiovascularly. As Allison says, "Any stroke will do!" That having been said, however, we do encourage you to develop proficiency in the basic strokes and to use them in your workout. Variety is the spice of life, and you'll get a more well-rounded workout.

Kickboard: In swimming, the kick is very important, but sometimes overlooked because the upper body does so much of the work in propulsion. A kickboard solves that problem and helps you develop the large muscles in your back, hips, and legs. The board is a small, flat, lightweight float that supports your weight in the water. You hang on with your hands, or wrap your arms around it, and use your legs alone to propel you.

Pull buoy: This is a flotation device you can loop around your shoulders to create drag as you swim. It makes the stroke a little harder for greater effort.

SWIMMING BEGINNER   1. Awakening the Body

DAY	1	Strength Work 2	3	Strength Work 4	5	Strength Work 6	7
WEEK 1 EASY	Make sure your clothing and equipment are in order.	Bob 5 min. Swim 10 min. Easy effort.	Bob 5 min. Swim 15 min. Easy effort.	Bob 5 min. Swim 10 min. Easy effort.	Rest.	Bob 5 min. Swim 10 min. Easy effort.	Bob 5 min. Swim 15 min. Easy effort.
2 MODERATE	Rest.	Bob 5 min. Kickboard 10 min. Easy effort.	Bob 5 min. Swim 15 min. Easy effort.	Rest.	Bob 5 min. Kickboard 10 min. Easy effort.	Rest.	Bob 5 min. Swim 15 min. Easy effort.
3 EASY							
4 HARD							
5 EASY							
6 HARD							

DAY	1	Strength Work 2	3	Strength Work 4	5	Strength Work 6	7
WEEK 1 EASY	Rest.	Bob 5 min. Swim 15 min. Easy effort.	Bob 5 min. Swim 10 min. Easy effort.	Bob 5 min. Swim 15 min. Easy effort.	Rest.	Bob 5 min. Swim 10 min. Easy effort.	Bob 5 min. Swim 15 min. Easy effort.
2 MODERATE	Rest.	Bob 5 min. Kickboard 10 min. Easy effort.	Bob 5 min. Swim 15 min. Easy effort.	Rest.	Bob 5 min. Kickboard 10 min. Easy effort.	Rest.	Bob 5 min. Kickboard 10 min. Easy effort.
3 EASY	Rest.	Bob 5 min. Swim 15 min. Easy effort.	Rest.	Bob 5 min. Swim 15 min. Easy effort.	Rest.	Bob 5 min. Swim 10 min. Easy effort.	Bob 5 min. Swim 15 min. Easy effort.
4 HARD	Rest.	Bob 5 min. Kickboard 5 min. Swim 10 min. Easy effort.	Bob 5 min. Swim 15 min. Easy effort.	Bob 5 min. Kickboard 5 min. Swim 10 min. Easy effort.	Rest.	Bob 5 min. Kickboard 5 min. Swim 10 min. Easy effort.	Bob 5 min. Swim 10 min. Easy effort.
5 EASY	Rest.	Bob 5 min. Swim 15 min. Easy effort.	Rest.	Rest.	Bob 5 min. Swim 15 min. Easy effort.	Rest.	Bob 5 min. Swim 10 min. Easy effort.
6 HARD	Rest.	Bob 5 min. Kickboard 5 min. Swim 10 min. Easy effort.	Bob 5 min. Kickboard 5 min. Swim 5 min. Easy effort.	Bob 5 min. Kickboard 5 min. Swim 10 min. Easy effort.	Rest.	Bob 5 min. Kickboard 5 min. Swim 10 min. Easy effort.	Bob 5 min. Kickboard 5 min. Swim 10 min. Easy effort.

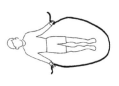

SWIMMING BEGINNER *2. Laying the Foundation*

SWIMMING BEGINNER   *3. Building Endurance*

DAY	1	Strength Work 2	3	Strength Work 4	5	Strength Work 6	7
WEEK 1 EASY	Rest.	Bob 5 min. Kickboard 5 min. Swim 10 min. Easy effort.	Bob 5 min. Swim 10 min. Easy effort.	Rest.	Bob 5 min. Swim 10 min. Easy effort.	Rest.	Bob 5 min. Kickboard 5 min. Swim 15 min. Easy effort.
2 MODERATE	Rest.	Bob 5 min. Kickboard 5 min. Swim 10 min. Easy effort.	Bob 5 min. Kickboard 5 min. Swim 15 min. Easy effort.	Bob 5 min. Kickboard 5 min. Swim 10 min. Easy effort.	Rest.	Bob 5 min. Kickboard 5 min. Swim 15 min. Easy effort.	Bob 5 min. Kickboard 10 min. Easy effort.
3 EASY	Rest.	Bob 5 min. Swim 15 min. Easy effort.	Bob 5 min. Kickboard 5 min. Swim 10 min. Easy effort.	Rest.	Bob 5 min. Swim 15 min. Easy effort.	Rest.	Bob 5 min. Kickboard 5 min. Swim 15 min. Easy effort.
4 HARD	Rest.	Bob 5 min. Kickboard 15 min. Easy effort.	Bob 5 min. Kickboard 10 min. Swim 10 min. Easy effort.	Bob 5 min. Kickboard 15 min. Easy effort.	Rest.	Bob 5 min. Kickboard 5 min. Swim 10 min. Easy effort.	Bob 5 min. Kickboard 15 min. Easy effort.
5 EASY	Rest.	Bob 5 min. Swim 20 min. Easy effort.	Bob 5 min. Kickboard 5 min. Swim 15 min. Easy effort.	Rest.	Bob 5 min. Swim 20 min. Easy effort.	Rest.	Bob 5 min. Kickboard 5 min. Swim 15 min. Easy effort.
6 HARD	Rest.	Bob 5 min. Kickboard 15 min. Swim 10 min. Easy effort.	Bob 5 min. Kickboard 5 min. Swim 10 min. Easy effort.	Bob 5 min. Kickboard 15 min. Swim 10 min. Easy effort.	Rest.	Bob 5 min. Kickboard 15 min. Swim 10 min. Easy effort.	Bob 5 min. Kickboard 15 min. Swim 15 min. Easy effort.

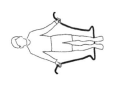

DAY	1	Strength Work 2	3	Strength Work 4	5	Strength Work 6	7
WEEK 1 EASY	Rest.	Bob 5 min. Swim 15 min. Easy effort.	Bob 5 min. Swim 20 min. Easy effort.	Rest.	Bob 5 min. Swim 15 min. Easy effort.	Bob 5 min. Swim 20 min. Easy effort.	Bob 5 min. Swim 15 min. Easy effort.
2 MODERATE	Rest.	Bob 5 min. Kickboard 10 min. Swim 15 min. Easy effort.	Bob 5 min. Kickboard 15 min. Swim 15 min. Easy effort.	Bob 5 min. Kickboard 10 min. Swim 15 min. Easy effort.	Rest.	Bob 5 min. Kickboard 10 min. Swim 15 min. Easy effort.	Bob 5 min. Kickboard 10 min. Swim 15 min. Easy effort.
3 EASY							
4 HARD							
5 EASY							
6 HARD							

SWIMMING BEGINNER *4. Achieving Mastery*

DAY	1	Strength Work 2	3	Strength Work 4	5	Strength Work 6	7
WEEK 1 EASY	Rest.	Bob 5 min. Swim 15 min. Easy effort.	Bob 5 min. Swim 20 min. Easy effort.	Bob 5 min. Swim 15 min. Easy effort.	Rest.	Bob 5 min. Swim 20 min. Easy effort.	Bob 5 min. Swim 15 min. Easy effort.
2 MODERATE	Rest.	Bob 5 min. Kickboard 15 min. Swim 10 min. Easy effort.	Bob 5 min. Kickboard 10 min. Swim 15 min. Easy effort.	Bob 5 min. Kickboard 15 min. Swim 10 min. Easy effort.	Rest.	Bob 5 min. Kickboard 10 min. Swim 15 min. Easy effort.	Bob 5 min. Kickboard 15 min. Swim 10 min. Easy effort.
3 EASY							
4 HARD							
5 EASY							
6 HARD							

SWIMMING INTERMEDIATE 5. Awakening the Body

DAY	1	Strength Work 2	3	Strength Work 4	5	Strength Work 6	7
WEEK 1 EASY	Rest.	Bob 5 min. Swim 15 min. Easy effort.	Bob 5 min. Swim 20 min. Easy effort.	Bob 5 min. Swim 15 min. Easy effort.	Rest.	Bob 5 min. Swim 15 min. Easy effort.	Bob 5 min. Swim 20 min. Easy effort.
2 MODERATE	Rest.	Bob 5 min. Kickboard 10 min. Swim 15 min. Easy effort.	Bob 5 min. Kickboard 5 min. Swim 15 min. Easy effort.	Bob 5 min. Kickboard 10 min. Swim 15 min. Easy effort.	Rest.	Bob 5 min. Kickboard 10 min. Swim 15 min. Easy effort.	Bob 5 min. Kickboard 10 min. Swim 20 min. Easy effort.
3 EASY	Rest.	Bob 5 min. Swim 15 min. Easy effort.	Rest.	Bob 5 min. Swim 15 min. Easy effort.	Rest.	Bob 5 min. Swim 15 min. Easy effort.	Bob 5 min. Swim 20 min. Easy effort.
4 HARD	Rest.	Bob 5 min. Kickboard 20 min. Easy effort.	Bob 5 min. Swim 20 min. Easy effort.	Bob 5 min. Kickboard 20 min. Easy effort.	Rest.	Bob 5 min. Kickboard 15 min. Swim 15 min. Easy effort.	Bob 5 min. Kickboard 20 min. Easy effort.
5 EASY	Rest.	Bob 5 min. Swim 15 min. Easy effort.	Rest.	Bob 5 min. Swim 15 min. Easy effort.	Rest.	Bob 5 min. Swim 15 min. Easy effort.	Bob 5 min. Swim 20 min. Easy effort.
6 HARD	Rest.	Bob 5 min. Kickboard 20 min. Moderate effort.	Bob 5 min. Swim 20 min. Moderate effort.	Bob 5 min. Kickboard 20 min. Moderate effort.	Rest.	Bob 5 min. Kickboard 15 min. Swim 20 min. Moderate effort.	Bob 5 min. Kickboard 20 min. Moderate effort.

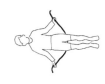

SWIMMING INTERMEDIATE 6. *Laying the Foundation*

SWIMMING INTERMEDIATE 7. Building Endurance

DAY	1	Strength Work 2	3	Strength Work 4	5	Strength Work 6	7
WEEK 1 EASY	Rest.	Bob 5 min. Swim 15 min. Moderate effort.	Bob 5 min. Swim 20 min. Moderate effort.	Bob 5 min. Swim 15 min. Moderate effort.	Rest.	Bob 5 min. Swim 20 min. Moderate effort.	Bob 5 min. Swim 20 min. Easy effort.
2 MODERATE	Rest.	Bob 5 min. Kickboard 10 min. Swim 15 min. Moderate effort.	Bob 5 min. Kickboard 15 min. Swim 10 min. Moderate effort.	Bob 5 min. Kickboard 10 min. Swim 15 min. Moderate effort.	Rest.	Bob 5 min. Kickboard 15 min. Swim 10 min. Moderate effort.	Bob 5 min. Kickboard 15 min. Swim 15 min. Moderate effort.
3 EASY	Rest.	Bob 5 min. Swim 20 min. Moderate effort.	Rest.	Bob 5 min. Swim 15 min. Moderate effort.	Rest.	Bob 5 min. Swim 20 min. Moderate effort.	Bob 5 min. Swim 20 min. Easy effort.
4 HARD	Rest.	Bob 5 min. Kickboard 20 min. Moderate effort.	Bob 5 min. Kickboard 15 min. Moderate effort.	Bob 5 min. Kickboard 15 min. Swim 15 min. Moderate effort.	Rest.	Bob 5 min. Kickboard 20 min. Swim 15 min. Moderate effort.	Bob 5 min. Kickboard 25 min. Easy effort.
5 EASY	Rest.	Bob 5 min. Swim 20 min. Easy effort.	Rest.	Bob 5 min. Swim 25 min. Easy effort.	Rest.	Bob 5 min. Swim 25 min. Easy effort.	Bob 5 min. Swim 20 min. Moderate effort.
6 HARD	Rest.	Bob 5 min. Kickboard 20 min. Swim 10 min. Moderate effort.	Bob 5 min. Kickboard 20 min. Swim 15 min. Moderate effort.	Bob 5 min. Kickboard 20 min. Swim 10 min. Moderate effort.	Rest.	Bob 5 min. Kickboard 25 min. Moderate effort.	Bob 5 min. Kickboard 30 min. Easy effort.

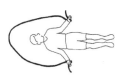

DAY	1	Strength Work 2	3	Strength Work 4	5	Strength Work 6	7
WEEK 1 EASY	Rest.	Bob 5 min. Swim 10 min. Moderate effort.	Bob 5 min. Swim 10 min. Moderate effort.	Bob 5 min. Kickboard 20 min. Swim 10 min. Moderate effort.	Rest.	Bob 5 min. Swim 20 min. Moderate effort.	Bob 5 min. Kickboard 20 min. Swim 10 min. Moderate effort.
2 MODERATE	Rest.	Bob 5 min. Kickboard 25 min. Moderate effort.	Bob 5 min. Kickboard 20 min. Moderate effort.	Bob 5 min. Kickboard 25 min. Moderate effort.	Rest.	Bob 5 min. Kickboard 20 min. Swim 10 min. Moderate effort.	Bob 5 min. Kickboard 25 min. Moderate effort.
3 EASY	Rest.	Bob 5 min. Swim 25 min. Moderate effort.	Rest.	Bob 5 min. Swim 20 min. Moderate effort.	Rest.	Bob 5 min. Swim 20 min. Moderate effort.	Bob 5 min. Swim 25 min. Moderate effort.
4 HARD	Rest.	Bob 5 min. Kickboard 20 min. Swim 20 min. Moderate effort.	Bob 5 min. Kickboard 20 min. Swim 15 min. Moderate effort.	Bob 5 min. Kickboard 20 min. Swim 20 min. Moderate effort.	Rest.	Bob 5 min. Kickboard 20 min. Swim 15 min. Moderate effort.	Bob 5 min. Kickboard 20 min. Swim 20 min. Moderate effort.
5 EASY							
6 HARD							

DAY	1	Strength Work 2	3	Strength Work 4	5	Strength Work 6	7
WEEK 1 EASY	Rest.	Bob 5 min. Kickboard 20 min. Swim 10 min. Moderate effort.	Bob 5 min. Swim 20 min. Moderate effort.	Bob 5 min. Swim 20 min. Hard effort.	Rest.	Bob 5 min. Kickboard 20 min. Swim 10 min. Moderate effort.	Bob 5 min. Swim 25 min. Moderate effort.
2 MODERATE	Rest.	Bob 5 min. Kickboard 20 min. Swim 10 min. Moderate effort.	Rest.	Bob 5 min. Kickboard 10 min. Swim 10 min. Hard effort.	Rest.	Bob 5 min. Kickboard 15 min. Swim 10 min. Moderate effort.	Bob 5 min. Kickboard 20 min. Swim 10 min. Hard effort.
3 EASY							
4 HARD							
5 EASY							
6 HARD							

SWIMMING ADVANCED   9. Awakening the Body

SWIMMING ADVANCED 10. Laying the Foundation

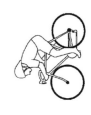

DAY	1	Strength Work 2	3	Strength Work 4	5	Strength Work 6	7
WEEK 1 EASY	Rest.	Bob 5 min. Swim 30 min. Moderate effort.	Bob 5 min. Swim 20 min. Hard effort.	Bob 5 min. Swim 30 min. Moderate effort.	Rest.	Bob 5 min. Kickboard 20 min. Swim 10 min. Hard effort.	Bob 5 min. Swim 30 min. Moderate effort.
2 MODERATE	Rest.	Bob 5 min. Kickboard 20 min. Swim 20 min. Hard effort.	Bob 5 min. Swim 30 min. Hard effort.	Bob 5 min. Kickboard 20 min. Swim 20 min. Hard effort.	Rest.	Bob 5 min. Kickboard 20 min. Swim 20 min. Hard effort.	Bob 5 min. Kickboard 20 min. Swim 20 min. Moderate effort.
3 EASY	Rest.	Bob 5 min. Swim 30 min. Hard effort.	Rest.	Bob 5 min. Swim 30 min. Moderate effort.	Rest.	Bob 5 min. Swim 30 min. Hard effort.	Bob 5 min. Swim 30 min. Moderate effort.
4 HARD	Rest.	Bob 5 min. Kickboard 20 min. Hard effort.	Bob 5 min. Kickboard 25 min. Hard effort.	Bob 5 min. Kickboard 20 min. Swim 10 min. Hard effort.	Rest.	Bob 5 min. Kickboard 30 min. Hard effort.	Bob 5 min. Kickboard 25 min. Swim 10 min. Hard effort.
5 EASY	Rest.	Bob 5 min. Kickboard 20 min. Swim 10 min. Hard effort.	Game Day.	Bob 5 min. Kickboard 20 min. Swim 10 min. Hard effort.	Rest.	Bob 5 min. Kickboard 20 min. Swim 10 min. Hard effort.	Bob 5 min. Swim 30 min. Hard effort.
6 HARD	Rest.	Bob 5 min. Kickboard 30 min. Swim 10 min. Hard effort.	Game Day.	Bob 5 min. Kickboard 30 min. Swim 10 min. Hard effort.	Rest.	Bob 5 min. Kickboard 35 min. Hard effort.	Bob 5 min. Kickboard 30 min. Swim 10 min. Hard effort.

DAY	1	2 Strength Work	3	4 Strength Work	5	6 Strength Work	7
WEEK 1 EASY	Rest.	Bob 5 min. Swim 35 min. Moderate effort.	Bob 5 min. Swim 25 min. Hard effort.	Bob 5 min. Swim 35 min. Moderate effort.	Rest.	Bob 5 min. Kickboard 20 min. Swim 20 min. Hard effort.	Bob 5 min. Swim 35 min. Moderate effort.
2 MODERATE	Rest.	Bob 5 min. Kickboard 30 min. Swim 10 min. Hard effort.	Bob 5 min. Swim 40 min. Hard effort.	Bob 5 min. Kickboard 25 min. Swim 20 min. Hard effort.	Rest.	Bob 5 min. Kickboard 25 min. Swim 20 min. Hard effort.	Bob 5 min. Kickboard 25 min. Swim 20 min. Moderate effort.
3 EASY	Rest.	Bob 5 min. Swim 35 min. Hard effort.	Rest.	Bob 5 min. Swim 35 min. Moderate effort.	Rest.	Bob 5 min. Swim 35 min. Hard effort.	Bob 5 min. Swim 40 min. Moderate effort.
4 HARD	Rest.	Bob 5 min. Kickboard 20 min. Swim 20 min. Hard effort.	Bob 5 min. Kickboard 25 min. Hard effort.	Bob 5 min. Kickboard 10 min. Swim 10 min. Hard effort. Add pull buoy.	Rest.	Bob 5 min. Kickboard 30 min. Swim 10 min. Hard effort.	Bob 5 min. Kickboard 25 min. Swim 10 min. Hard effort. Add pull buoy.
5 EASY	Rest.	Bob 5 min. Kickboard 20 min. Swim 10 min. Hard effort. Add pull buoy.	Game Day.	Bob 5 min. Kickboard 20 min. Swim 10 min. Hard effort. Add pull buoy.	Rest.	Bob 5 min. Kickboard 20 min. Swim 10 min. Hard effort. Add pull buoy.	Bob 5 min. Swim 30 min. Hard effort. Add pull buoy.
6 HARD	Rest.	Bob 5 min. Kickboard 30 min. Swim 10 min. Hard effort. Add pull buoy.	Game Day.	Bob 5 min. Kickboard 30 min. Swim 10 min. Hard effort. Add pull buoy.	Rest.	Bob 5 min. Kickboard 35 min. Hard effort.	Bob 5 min. Kickboard 30 min. Swim 10 min. Hard effort. Add pull buoy.

SWIMMING ADVANCED   *11. Building Endurance*

DAY	1	Strength Work 2	3	Strength Work 4	5	Strength Work 6	7
WEEK 1 EASY	Rest.	Bob 5 min. Swim 20 min. Hard effort. Add pull buoy.	Bob 5 min. Swim 25 min. Hard effort. Add pull buoy.	Game Day.	Rest.	Bob 5 min. Swim 20 min. Hard effort. Add pull buoy.	Bob 5 min. Kickboard 20 min. Swim 10 min. Hard effort. Add pull buoy.
2 MODERATE	Rest.	Bob 5 min. Kickboard 30 min. Swim 10 min. Hard effort. Add pull buoy.	Bob 5 min. Kickboard 35 min. Swim 10 min. Hard effort. Add pull buoy.	Game Day.	Rest.	Bob 5 min. Kickboard 35 min. Swim 10 min. Hard effort. Add pull buoy.	Bob 5 min. Kickboard 40 min. Swim 10 min. Hard effort. Add pull buoy.
3 EASY	Rest.	Bob 5 min. Kickboard 10 min. Swim 30 min. Hard effort. Add pull buoy.	Bob 5 min. Kickboard 10 min. Swim 35 min. Hard effort. Add pull buoy.	Game Day.	Rest.	Bob 5 min. Kickboard 10 min. Swim 35 min. Hard effort. Add pull buoy.	Bob 5 min. Kickboard 10 min. Swim 25 min. Hard effort. Add pull buoy.
4 HARD	Rest.	Bob 5 min. Swim 35 min. Hard effort.	Bob 5 min. Swim 50 min. Moderate effort.	Bob 5 min. Swim 45 min. Moderate effort.	Rest.	Bob 5 min. Swim 55 min. Moderate effort.	Bob 5 min. Swim 60 min. Moderate effort.
5 EASY							
6 HARD							

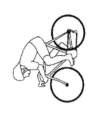

SWIMMING ADVANCED 12. Achieving Mastery

IN-LINE SKATING

See art, pages 67–99.

TECHNIQUE AND FORM

No question about it, in-line skating is a dream come true for an athlete in search of a program. It provides low-impact aerobic exercise, can be done almost anywhere, requires inexpensive basic equipment, and is loads of fun.

In-line skating starts with balance and coordination. Because the basic building block of in-line skating is the move forward on the pavement, you begin by pushing off. One foot stabilizes at a slight angle. You press your weight against that foot while you run the other foot forward at an opposite angle. You shift your weight over the advanced foot and begin the process all over again. In stabilizing, you use the abductors in your hips, buttocks (gluteals), thighs (quads), and calves (soleus). You flex your trunk forward, engaging your abdominals, lower back, and hip flexors and extensors to create forward thrust. For turns, you'll rely on your hip abductors and adductors. For spins, you'll use your hip and trunk rotators. For jumps, you'll stress your gluteals and abdominals. For backward movement, you'll engage neck rotators, hyperextend your hip for direction changes, and abduct and adduct your hips for propulsion. Arm and torso swinging (rhythmic side to side motion) is controlled by your hip rotators, abductors, and adductors, with your back and abdominals providing stabilization.

In-line skating is now designated an "extreme" sport. It earned its reputation by combining speed, aerobics, and acrobatics into gravity-defying choreography that can, at times, threaten life and limb. An athlete who takes the sport to the extreme is called an "aggro," meaning he or she is an aggressive skater. Although we *all* have moments when we think of ourselves as aggros, most of us, most of the time, fall (no pun intended) into a range a little less aggro and a little more earthbound.

It's no wonder that in-line skating is enjoying such rampant popularity. It's fun and uncomplicated. To participate requires one skater, one pair of skates, protective equipment, and a stretch of pavement. (Unless you're an aggro. Then you need to add railings, steps, vaults, ramps, culverts, and an insurance agent with a sense of humor.)

EQUIPMENT YOU'LL NEED

A watch

A bottle of water

An identification card to put into your pocket

Cell phone (perhaps in a fanny pack)

Skates

Helmet

Elbow, wrist, knee protectors

Padded gloves

Repair kit with tools

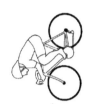

WHAT TO WEAR

Skates: Selecting the right skates is an important component to your success in the sport. You get what you pay for. We recommend that you talk to experienced skaters, study the magazine reviews, and then shop in a store with staff who specialize in skates and fitting them. (If you can, rent skates to have some basis for decisions about features you like and don't like.)

Make sure the boot is snug, but comfortable. It has to support your foot and ankle, yet give you room for your toes. The cuff of the boot should cover your ankle bone completely and give you plenty of lateral support so that the side-to-side movement of your ankle is restricted. Make sure the liner is soft and comfortable. The fastening system of the boot will vary by manufacturer, and is a matter of preference. You can choose either laces, which allow you to fine-tune the fit, or buckles, which allow you the convenience and fit of a ski boot.

Selecting the frames, bearings, and wheels is tricky. Designs and materials vary according to use. No matter what you choose, make sure the equipment is durable and will give you solid, smooth roll.

The brakes are critical. There are several systems now being manufactured, with daily advances in technology. Don't leave the store before you understand how they work and have a good feel for the action. (Note: before you get too far into your training, make sure you learn to T-stop without brakes, just in case they fail.)

Clothing: Wear clothing that is appropriate for the weather, and is loose and comfortable so you can move easily. Many skaters wear long-sleeved shirts and long pants to minimize scrapes in the case of a fall, but this choice is personal. Some skaters wear padded shorts that cushion a blow when they land on their backsides. Wear whatever makes you feel great.

Socks: Look for a smooth, snug fit that's free from wrinkles and inside seams. Most skaters prefer a sort of tube sock that protects all the way up the shin beyond the top of the boot; a sock that stops short might cause irritations. Because even the best socks are an inexpensive investment, go first-class. Purchase athletes' socks that are engineered to wick moisture, or absorb sweat away from your foot and provide you with a dryer boot interior, which will help prevent blistering, skin irritations, and odor. Treat yourself to a clean pair of socks with every workout.

BOREDOM BUSTERS

Listen to music: Portable CD and tape players, and radios with lightweight headsets, are popular among skaters. After all, much of in-line skating is dancing. If you're skating in the company of other people, be sure you're using a headset that affords you complete privacy. In other words, do everything possible to keep from imposing (or inflicting) your choice of music—and its accompanying rhythms—on other skaters. When using a headset, leave one ear totally free so that you can hear what's going on around you and stay alert to your environment. If you are skating beside a roadway, leave free the ear that is closest to traffic. Digital stereo is great, but it's dangerous in a workout.

Recruit a partner: For athletes who train outside on streets or on sidewalks, there's safety in numbers. There's also motivation. You and a friend can work together to keep your training schedules on track. Better yet, join a club or a skating group where you can work out with other skaters.

Play utility poles: This game is a favorite of runners, to introduce speed work, or "tempo," into training, but it adapts very well to in-line skating. Utility poles are good gauges of precise distance because they are evenly placed beside the road. Pick up your pace from the first pole to the second, then back off until you reach the third pole. Step up your pace again, and so on. As you develop stamina, try increasing the numbers of poles between which you pick up your pace, such as picking up the pace for three poles, then backing off for one pole.

Get extreme: Your training schedule for in-line skating is pretty straightforward, but the truth is that the sport offers amazing opportunities for dance, acrobatics, and aerobatics. Mix it up a little. We're not telling you to get crazy and put your life on the line, but we are telling you that you don't want to miss out on the fun. Find a good teacher (like an eleven-year-old with the look of a veteran) and try a few moves.

Set up cones: You can buy inexpensive traffic control cones from any good hardware or automotive-supply store. Get a few and set up an obstacle course that will help you sharpen your agility and reflexes.

Take yourself to a skate park: For a little adventure and challenge, take your skates to a recreational facility especially developed for in-line skating. You'll find trails, pipes, jumps, and bowls designed for perfect skate physics. Unlike the sidewalks and roads to which you are accustomed, here the surfaces are smooth and uncluttered. Not only will you have a great time, but the staff and other skaters can give you some pointers that might improve your skating.

TAKING IT TO THE GYM
Slide mat and booties

INJURY ALERT

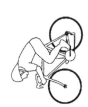

We said earlier that in-line skating was a low-impact sport. We sort of lied. It can be a huge-impact sport . . . especially when a face meets the pavement. In this sport, most injuries are traumatic: those that take place when a skater falls or slams into something. Skaters are also prone to overuse and chronic injuries such as tendinitis. Experts advise that injuries involving trauma can be mitigated with the use of protective equipment such as wrist and knee guards, and the all-important helmet. We mean it—wear it!

Literature on in-line skating is loaded with admonishments to closely monitor the surface on which you skate. Look for holes, ridges, bumps, and debris. Be especially vigilant if you change the time of day (or night) when you skate, because light transforms the way surfaces look. A demon ridge that casts a long shadow at five o'clock in the afternoon may disappear altogether at high noon. And if you are skating in a group, be considerate. When you spot an obstacle, call it out for those who are skating behind you. Oh, yes, and skate around it.

TIPS FROM THE EXPERTS

Non-negotiable Wharton rule: don't strap on the first skate before putting on *all* your protective equipment.

When you skate, remember that you're silent and fast. Be careful when you're skating around other people. One unexpected move by someone who doesn't see you coming, and you could collide.

In-line skating is a wonderful aerobic workout that lets you work your lower extremities, but your upper body is neglected. You'll want to supplement your training with general strength and flexibility work, upper-body work, and a little extra leg- and footwork. Your skate boot restricts your foot and ankle movement, and prevents your legs from getting a complete, well-balanced workout.

Please remember to hydrate. In-line skating is a strenuous, demanding sport in both training and competition. Even slight dehydration lowers the circulating volume of blood and causes the core temperature to rise. Symptoms of progressive dehydration include fatigue, lack of coordination, muscle pain and cramping, headache, light-headedness, confusion, disorientation, and fainting. Under extreme circumstances, death can occur. If you feel thirsty, you're already on your way to trouble. Drink early—before thirst sets in—and often. Experts say that water is perfect for short workouts, but a commercial sport fluid-replacement drink is preferable for workouts of more than ninety minutes in duration. With either choice, *cold* is best. We want you to play it cool. Drink.

COMING TO TERMS WITH THE TERMS WE USE IN YOUR SCHEDULE

Skate: This is a leisurely, conversational pace. You should be in the minimum range of your target heart rate. We want you to concentrate on perfect form and get used to your shoes.

Stride out: This is a quickened pace, but still conversational. You should be in the middle to upper-middle range of your target heart rate.

Sprint: This is race pace. You'll be exerting effort. You should be in the higher ranges of your target heart rate.

Normal pace: You'll find this reference in the beginning to remind you to stay under control.

Pick up the pace: For a short duration, put extra effort into your workout. Literally, pick it up.

Surfaces: If we specify the topography (such as rolling hills or flat surfaces), do your best to follow our suggestions. If working out on specific surfaces isn't possible, any surface will do. If we haven't specified a surface, choose one you like.

Skating form: You'll notice we did not specify skills and maneuvers. In working out, what you do is less important than the time and effort you put into the activity. We do, however, encourage you to become proficient at skating; a good coach can help. Not only will your workouts be more interesting, but you'll enjoy the complexities and challenge of your sport.

IN-LINE SKATING BEGINNER   1. Awakening the Body

DAY	1	Strength Work 2	3	Strength Work 4	5	Strength Work 6	7
WEEK 1 EASY	Make sure your skates and protective equipment are in order.	Skate 15 min. on flat surface.	Skate 15 min. on flat surface.	Skate 15 min. Pick up the pace.	Rest.	Skate 5 min. at normal pace. Skate 15 min. Pick up the pace.	Skate 5 min. at normal pace. Skate 15 min. Pick up the pace.
2 MODERATE	Rest.	Skate 5 min. Stride out 5 min. (Easy does it!) Skate 5 min.	Skate 15 min. on flat surface.	Rest.	Skate 5 min. Stride out 5 min. (Easy does it!) Skate 5 min.	Rest.	Skate 5 min. at normal pace. Skate 15 min. Pick up the pace.
3 EASY							
4 HARD							
5 EASY							
6 HARD							

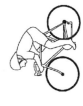

10. The Ten Best Cardio-Fit Activities and Training Schedules   **173**

IN-LINE SKATING BEGINNER   *2. Laying the Foundation*

	DAY 1	Strength Work 2	3	Strength Work 4	5	Strength Work 6	7
WEEK 1 EASY	Rest.	Skate 20 min.	Skate 5 min. Skate/Stride out 20 min. (alternate skating and striding in 5-min. intervals). Skate 5 min.	Skate 20 min.	Rest.	Skate 20 min.	Skate 5 min. Skate/Stride out 10 min. (alternate skating and striding in 5-min. intervals). Skate 5 min.
2 MODERATE	Rest.	Skate 10 min. Stride out 20 min. Skate 10 min.	Skate 20 min. on flat surface.	Rest.	Skate 5 min. Skate/Stride out 10 min. (alternate skating and striding in 5-min. intervals). Skate 5 min.	Rest.	Skate 10 min. Stride out 5 min. Skate 10 min.
3 EASY	Rest.	Skate 25 min. on flat surface.	Rest.	Skate 25 min.	Rest.	Skate 5 min. Stride out 20 min.	Skate 5 min. Stride out 5 min. Skate 5 min. Stride out 5 min. Skate 5 min.
4 HARD	Rest.	Skate 5 min. Stride out 5 min. Skate 5 min. Stride out 5 min. Skate 5 min.	Stride out 25 min. Skate 5 min.	Skate 5 min. Stride out 5 min. Skate 5 min.	Rest.	Skate 20 min.	Skate 30 min.
5 EASY	Rest.	Skate 5 min. Stride out 10 min. Skate 5 min. Stride out 5 min. Skate 5 min.	Rest.	Rest.	Skate 5 min. Skate/Stride out 10 min. (alternate skating and striding in 1-min. intervals). Skate 10 min.	Rest.	Skate 5 min. Stride out 10 min. Skate 10 min.
6 HARD	Rest.	Skate 30 min.	Skate 5 min. Stride out 15 min. Skate 5 min.	Skate 10 min. Stride out 5 min. Skate 10 min.	Rest.	Skate 20 min.	Skate 5 min. Stride out 10 min. Skate 10 min.

DAY	1	Strength Work 2	3	Strength Work 4	5	Strength Work 6	7
WEEK 1 EASY	Rest.	Rolling hill work: Skate 5 min. Stride out 5 min. Skate 5 min.	Skate 5 min. Stride out 10 min. Skate 5 min.	Rest.	Rolling hill work: Skate 5 min. Stride out 10 min. Skate 5 min. Skate 5 min.	Rest.	Skate 5 min. Stride out 20 min. Skate 5 min.
2 MODERATE	Rest.	Rolling hill work: Skate 5 min. Stride out 10 min. Skate 5 min.	Stride out 5 min. Sprint 10 min. Stride out 5 min.	Skate 10 min. Stride out 10 min. Skate 10 min.	Rest.	Skate 5 min. Stride out 15 min. Skate 10 min.	Skate 5 min. Stride out 20 min. Skate 5 min.
3 EASY	Rest.	Rolling hill work: Skate 5 min. Stride out 10 min. Stride out 10 min. Skate 5 min.	Stride out 5 min. Sprint 15 min. Stride out 5 min.	Rest.	Rolling hill work: Skate 15 min. Stride out 15 min. Skate 10 min.	Rest.	Stride out 15 min. Sprint 20 min. Stride out 5 min.
4 HARD	Rest.	Rolling hill work: Skate 5 min. Stride out 20 min. Skate 5 min.	Stride out 5 min. Sprint 15 min. Stride out 5 min.	Rolling hill work: Skate 5 min. Stride out 5 min. Skate 5 min. Stride out 10 min. Skate 5 min.	Rest.	Skate 5 min. Stride out 20 min. Skate 5 min. Skate 5 min.	Stride out 15 min. Sprint 25 min. Stride out 5 min.
5 EASY	Rest.	Rolling hill work: Skate 5 min. Stride out 15 min. Skate 5 min. Stride out 10 min. Skate 5 min.	Stride out 5 min. Sprint 20 min. Stride out 5 min.	Rest.	Rolling hill work: Skate 5 min. Stride out 10 min. Skate 5 min. Stride out 5 min. Skate 5 min.	Rest.	Stride out 25 min.
6 HARD	Rest.	Rolling hill work: Skate 5 min. Stride out 10 min. Skate 5 min. Stride out 15 min. Skate 5 min.	Skate 5 min. Stride out 25 min. Skate 5 min.	Skate 5 min. Stride out 5 min. Skate 5 min. Stride out 20 min. Skate 5 min.	Rest.	Stride out 5 min. Sprint 10 min. Stride out 5 min.	Stride out 30 min.

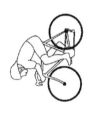

DAY		Strength Work			Strength Work			Strength Work	
WEEK	1	2	3	4	5	6	7
1 EASY	Rest.	Rolling hill work: Stride out 5 min. Sprint 25 min. Stride out 5 min.	Stride out 5 min. Sprint 15 min. Stride out 5 min. Sprint 10 min. Stride out 5 min.	Rest.	Rolling hill work: Stride out 5 min. Sprint 5 min. Stride out 5 min. Repeat entire pattern.	Stride out 5 min. Sprint 20 min. Stride out 5 min.	Stride out 5 min. Sprint 25 min. Stride out 5 min.
2 MODERATE	Rest.	Rolling hill work: Stride out 5 min. Sprint 25 min. Stride out 5 min.	Stride out 5 min. Sprint 10 min. Stride out 5 min. Sprint 10 min. Stride out 5 min.	Rolling hill work: Stride out 5 min. Sprint 15 min. Stride out 5 min. Sprint 10 min. Stride out 5 min.	Rest.	Rolling hill work: Stride out 10 min. Sprint 15 min. Stride out 5 min.	Stride out 20 min. Sprint 10 min. Stride out 10 min.
3 EASY							
4 HARD							
5 EASY							
6 HARD							

IN-LINE SKATING BEGINNER *4. Achieving Mastery*

DAY	1	Strength Work 2	3	Strength Work 4	5	Strength Work 6	7
WEEK 1 EASY	Rest.	On flat surface: Stride out 5 min. Sprint 25 min. Stride out 5 min.	Stride out 5 min. Sprint 10 min. Stride out 5 min. Sprint 10 min. Stride out 5 min.	Rolling hill work: Stride out 5 min. Sprint 15 min. Stride out 5 min. Sprint 10 min. Stride out 5 min.	Rest.	Rolling hill work: Stride out 10 min. Sprint 15 min. Stride out 5 min.	Rolling hill work: Stride out 20 min. Sprint 10 min. Stride out 10 min.
2 MODERATE	Rest.	Rolling hill work: Stride out 10 min. Sprint 25 min. Stride out 10 min.	Stride out 5 min. Sprint 15 min. Stride out 5 min. Sprint 15 min. Stride out 5 min.	Rolling hill work: Stride out 10 min. For 30 min., alternate 1 min. sprinting with 1 min. striding. Stride out 5 min.	Rest.	Rolling hill work: Stride out 10 min. Sprint 20 min. Stride out 5 min.	Stride out 10 min. Sprint 20 min. Stride out 5 min.
3 EASY							
4 HARD							
5 EASY							
6 HARD							

IN-LINE SKATING INTERMEDIATE   5. Awakening the Body

DAY	1	Strength Work 2	3	Strength Work 4	5	Strength Work 6	7
WEEK 1 EASY	Rest.	Rolling hill work: Stride out 30 min.	Stride out 5 min. Sprint 15 min. Stride out 5 min. Sprint 15 min. Stride out 5 min.	Rolling hill work: Stride out 10 min. For 25 min., alternate 1 min. striding with 1 min. sprinting. Stride out 5 min.	Rest.	Rolling hill work: Stride out 10 min. Sprint 20 min. Stride out 5 min.	Rolling hill work: Stride out 10 min. Sprint 20 min. Stride out 5 min.
2 MODERATE	Rest.	Rolling hill work: Stride out 20 min. Sprint 10 min. Stride out 5 min.	On flat surface: Stride out 5 min. Sprint 20 min. Stride out 5 min. Sprint 10 min. Stride out 5 min.	Rolling hill work: Stride out 5 min. For 35 min., alternate 5 min. striding with 5 min. sprinting. Stride out 5 min.	Rest.	Rolling hill work: Stride out 5 min. Sprint 25 min. Stride out 5 min.	Rolling hill work: Stride out 10 min. Sprint 20 min. Stride out 5 min.
3 EASY	Rest.	Rolling hill work: Stride out 15 min. Sprint 10 min. Stride out 5 min.	Stride out 5 min. Sprint 15 min. Stride out 5 min. Sprint 10 min. Stride out 5 min.	Rolling hill work: Stride out 5 min. For 35 min., alternate 5 min. striding with 5 min. sprinting. Stride out 5 min.	Rest.	Rolling hill work: Stride out 35 min.	Rolling hill work: Stride out 10 min. Sprint 20 min. Stride out 5 min.
4 HARD	Rest.	Rolling hill work: Stride out 30 min. Sprint 15 min. Stride out 5 min.	Stride out 5 min. Sprint 20 min. Stride out 5 min. Stride out 5 min.	Rolling hill work: Stride out 5 min. For 35 min., alternate 1 min. striding with 1 min. sprinting. Stride out 5 min.	Rest.	Rolling hill work: Sprint 25 min. Stride out 5 min.	Rolling hill work: Stride out 10 min. Sprint 20 min. Stride out 5 min.
5 EASY	Rest.	Rolling hill work: Stride out 10 min. Sprint 10 min. Stride out 5 min.	Stride out 10 min. Sprint 10 min. Stride out 5 min. Sprint 5 min. Stride out 5 min.	Rolling hill work: Stride out 5 min. For 35 min., alternate 5 min. striding with 5 min. sprinting. Stride out 5 min.	Rest.	Rolling hill work: Stride out 5 min. Sprint 25 min. Stride out 5 min.	Rolling hill work: Stride out 10 min. Sprint 20 min. Stride out 5 min. Stride out 5 min.
6 HARD	Rest.	Rolling hill work: Stride out 10 min. Sprint 20 min. Stride out 5 min.	Stride out 10 min. Sprint 20 min. Stride out 5 min. Sprint 5 min. Stride out 5 min.	Rolling hill work: Stride out 5 min. For 35 min., alternate 5 min. striding with 5 min. sprinting. Stride out 5 min.	Rest.	Rolling hill work: Sprint 30 min. Stride out 5 min.	Rolling hill work: Stride out 10 min. Sprint 20 min. Stride out 5 min. Stride out 5 min.

IN-LINE SKATING INTERMEDIATE   6. Laying the Foundation

IN-LINE SKATING INTERMEDIATE 7. Building Endurance

DAY	1	Strength Work 2	3	4	5	Strength Work 6	7
WEEK 1 EASY	Rest.	Rolling hill work: Sprint 15 min. Stride out 5 min.	Rolling hill work: Stride out 10 min. Sprint 10 min. Stride out 5 min.	Rolling hill work: Sprint 5 min. Stride out 2 min. Sprint 5 min. Stride out 5 min.	Rest.	Stride out 20 min. Sprint 5 min. Stride out 5 min.	Rolling hill work: Stride out 30 min.
2 MODERATE	Rest.	Rolling hill work: Sprint 15 min. Stride out 5 min.	Rolling hill work: Stride out 10 min. Sprint 10 min. Stride out 5 min.	Rolling hill work: Sprint 5 min. Stride out 2 min. Sprint 10 min. Stride out 5 min.	Rest.	Stride out 15 min. Sprint 10 min. Stride out 5 min.	Rolling hill work: Sprint 30 min.
3 EASY	Rest.	Rolling hill work: Sprint 15 min. Stride out 5 min.	Rolling hill work: Stride out 15 min. Sprint 10 min. Stride out 5 min.	Rolling hill work: Sprint 5 min. Stride out 2 min. Sprint 5 min. Stride out 5 min.	Rest.	Stride out 20 min. Sprint 5 min. Stride out 5 min.	Rolling hill work: Sprint 30 min.
4 HARD	Rest.	Rolling hill work: Sprint 20 min. Stride out 5 min.	Rolling hill work: Stride out 15 min. Sprint 10 min. Stride out 5 min.	Rolling hill work: Sprint 5 min. Stride out 2 min. Sprint 7 min. Stride out 5 min.	Rest.	Stride out 20 min. Sprint 10 min. Stride out 5 min.	Rolling hill work: Sprint 30 min.
5 EASY	Rest.	Rolling hill work: Sprint 20 min. Stride out 5 min.	Rolling hill work: Stride out 15 min. Sprint 10 min. Stride out 5 min.	Rolling hill work: Sprint 5 min. Stride out 2 min. Sprint 7 min. Stride out 5 min.	Rest.	Stride out 20 min. Sprint 10 min. Stride out 5 min.	Rolling hill work: Sprint 35 min.
6 HARD	Rest.	Rolling hill work: Sprint 25 min. Stride out 5 min.	Rest.	Rolling hill work: Sprint 10 min. Stride out 2 min. Sprint 10 min. Stride out 5 min.	Rest.	Stride out 30 min.	Rolling hill work: Sprint 35 min.

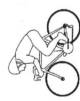

DAY	1	Strength Work 2	3	Strength Work 4	5	Strength Work 6	7
WEEK 1 EASY	Rest.	Rolling hill work: Sprint 35 min.	Rolling hill work: Stride out 5 min. Sprint 5 min. Stride out 5 min. Sprint 7 min. Stride out 5 min.	Rolling hill work: Stride out 10 min. Sprint 10 min. Stride out 10 min.	Rest.	Stride out 15 min. Sprint 10 min. Stride out 2 min.	Rolling hill work: Sprint 35 min. Stride out 5 min.
2 MODERATE	Rest.	Rolling hill work: Sprint 35 min.	Rolling hill work: Stride out 5 min. Sprint 10 min. Stride out 5 min. Sprint 7 min. Stride out 5 min.	Rolling hill work: Sprint 25 min. Stride out 5 min.	Rest.	Stride out 20 min. Sprint 10 min. Stride out 2 min.	Rolling hill work: Sprint 35 min. Stride out 5 min.
3 EASY	Rest.	Rolling hill work: Sprint 35 min.	Rest.	Rolling hill work: Sprint 20 min. Stride out 5 min.	Rest.	Stride out 15 min. Sprint 10 min. Stride out 2 min.	Rolling hill work: Sprint 35 min. Stride out 5 min.
4 HARD	Rest.	Rolling hill work: Sprint 35 min.	Rolling hill work: Sprint 20 min. Stride out 5 min.	Rolling hill work: Sprint 25 min. Stride out 5 min.	Rest.	Stride out 10 min. Sprint 20 min. Stride out 2 min.	Rolling hill work: Sprint 35 min. Stride out 5 min.
5 EASY							
6 HARD							

IN-LINE SKATING INTERMEDIATE   *8. Achieving Mastery*

IN-LINE SKATING ADVANCED

DAY	1	Strength Work 2	3	Strength Work 4	5	Strength Work 6	7
WEEK 1 EASY	Rest.	Rolling hill work: Sprint 25 min. Stride out 5 min.	Stride out 10 min. Sprint 20 min. Stride out 5 min.	Stride out 5 min. Sprint 15 min. Stride out 10 min.	Rest.	Stride out 20 min. Sprint 20 min. Stride out 5 min.	Rolling hill work: Sprint 45 min. Stride out 5 min.
2 MODERATE	Rest.	Rolling hill work: Sprint 30 min. Stride out 5 min.	Rest.	Rolling hill work: Sprint 25 min. Stride out 5 min.	Rest.	Stride out 40 min.	Rolling hill work: Sprint 45 min. Stride out 5 min.
3 EASY							
4 HARD							
5 EASY							
6 HARD							

9. Awakening the Body

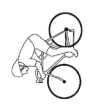

DAY	1	Strength Work 2	3	Strength Work 4	5	Strength Work 6	7
WEEK 1 EASY	Rest.	Rolling hill work: Sprint 35 min. Stride out 5 min.	Rolling hill work: Stride out 5 min. Sprint 30 min. Stride out 5 min.	Stride out 15 min. Sprint 10 min. Stride out 5 min.	Rest.	Stride out 20 min. Sprint 20 min.	Rolling hill work: Sprint 40 min. Stride out 5 min.
2 MODERATE	Rest.	Rolling hill work: Sprint 35 min. Stride out 5 min.	Rolling hill work: Stride out 5 min. Sprint 40 min. Stride out 5 min.	Stride out 20 min. Sprint 10 min. Stride out 5 min.	Rest.	Sprint 40 min.	Rolling hill work: Sprint 40 min. Stride out 5 min.
3 EASY	Rest.	Rolling hill work: Sprint 35 min. Stride out 5 min.	Rest.	Stride out 20 min. Sprint 10 min. Stride out 5 min.	Rest.	Stride out 20 min. Sprint 30 min.	Rolling hill work: Sprint 40 min. Stride out 5 min.
4 HARD	Rest.	Rolling hill work: Sprint 35 min. Stride out 5 min.	Rolling hill work: Stride out 5 min. Sprint 40 min. Stride out 5 min.	Stride out 25 min. Sprint 15 min. Stride out 5 min.	Rest.	Stride out 10 min. Sprint 20 min.	Rolling hill work: Sprint 40 min. Stride out 5 min.
5 EASY	Rest.	Rolling hill work: Sprint 35 min. Stride out 5 min.	Game Day.	Stride out 20 min. Sprint 20 min.	Rest.	Stride out 20 min. Sprint 20 min.	Rolling hill work: Sprint 40 min. Stride out 5 min.
6 HARD	Rest.	Rolling hill work: Sprint 35 min. Stride out 5 min.	Game Day.	Stride out 15 min. Sprint 30 min.	Rest.	Stride out 20 min. Sprint 20 min.	Rolling hill work: Sprint 40 min. Stride out 5 min.

IN-LINE SKATING ADVANCED   *10. Laying the Foundation*

IN-LINE SKATING ADVANCED   *11. Building Endurance*

DAY / WEEK	1	Strength Work 2	3	Strength Work 4	5	Strength Work 6	7
1 EASY	Rest.	Sprint 35 min. Keep a steady pace.	Game Day.	Stride out 10 min. Sprint 30 min. Stride out 5 min.	Rest.	Stride out 20 min. Sprint 20 min.	Sprint 45 min. Keep a steady pace.
2 MODERATE	Rest.	Sprint 40 min. Keep a steady pace.	Game Day.	Stride out 5 min. Sprint 40 min. Stride out 5 min.	Rest.	Stride out 20 min. Sprint 20 min.	Sprint 45 min. Keep a steady pace.
3 EASY	Rest.	Sprint 35 min. Keep a steady pace.	Game Day.	Sprint 45 min. Stride out 5 min.	Rest.	Stride out 20 min. Sprint 20 min.	Sprint 45 min. Keep a steady pace.
4 HARD	Rest.	Sprint 45 min. Keep a steady pace.	Game Day.	Sprint 45 min. Stride out 5 min.	Rest.	Stride out 20 min. Sprint 20 min.	Sprint 50 min. Keep a steady pace.
5 EASY	Rest.	Stride out 5 min. Sprint 15 min. Stride out 5 min. Sprint 15 min. Stride out 5 min.	Sprint 40 min. Keep a steady pace.	Game Day.	Rest.	Sprint 30 min. Keep a steady pace.	Sprint 45 min. Keep a steady pace.
6 HARD	Rest.	Stride out 5 min. Sprint 20 min. Stride out 5 min. Sprint 20 min. Stride out 5 min.	Sprint 45 min. Keep a steady pace.	Game Day.	Rest.	Sprint 30 min. Keep a steady pace.	Sprint 50 min. Keep a steady pace.

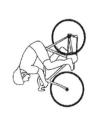

DAY	1	Strength Work 2	3	Strength Work 4	5	Strength Work 6	7
WEEK 1 EASY	Rest.	Stride out 5 min. Sprint 20 min. Stride out 5 min. Sprint 10 min. Stride out 5 min.	Sprint 40 min.	Game Day.	Rest.	Sprint 30 min.	Sprint 45 min.
2 MODERATE	Rest.	Stride out 5 min. Sprint 25 min. Stride out 5 min. Sprint 5 min. Stride out 5 min.	Sprint 50 min.	Game Day.	Rest.	Sprint 30 min.	Sprint 55 min.
3 EASY	Rest.	Stride out 5 min. Sprint 35 min. Stride out 10 min.	Sprint 30 min.	Game Day.	Rest.	Sprint 30 min.	Sprint 40 min.
4 HARD	Rest.	Sprint 35 min.	Sprint 40 min.	Sprint 30 min.	Rest.	Sprint 30 min.	Sprint 60 min.
5 EASY							
6 HARD							

IN-LINE SKATING ADVANCED   *12. Achieving Mastery*

CROSS-COUNTRY SKIING

See art, pages 269–287.

TECHNIQUE AND FORM

One of the handy things about cross-country skiing is that it's an outdoor sport that can be brought indoors. (Don't try this with downhill or jumping!) There are a number of good ski-track machines on the market that simulate the action of cross-country skiing. The one we have in our clinic is a big favorite of clients who want quick, effective cardiovascular workouts, and athletes with injuries that preclude impact to feet, legs, and hips. You lock your feet into narrow, sliding, parallel rails, turn on the CD player, slip on your heart monitor, set your timer, calibrate your resistance, grasp the handles of the arm pulleys, shout, "Mush, you huskies!" and take off. The machines are inexpensive, quiet, lightweight, easily stored, and provide a rather impressive workout.

As with all sports, however, we prefer that you take cross-country outside where you'll have more opportunity to . . . uh . . . cross some country. While ski-track machines lock you into a narrow range of motion, real skiing puts your whole body to work as you maneuver, turn, and handle uphill, downhill, and everything else in between. There is also much to be said for fresh air, sunshine, and a snowy trail with your name on it.

Cross-country skiing is a highly technical and physically demanding sport and one that can't be learned from a book (and certainly not this page). Because it involves snow, speed, uneven terrain, slick skis, and unyielding pine trees, it's imperative that you learn from the best, most experienced instructor you can find. If you can't afford a private instructor, almost all ski resorts offer inexpensive group classes, where you can enjoy the camaraderie of other skiers while you learn.

Basic, or "classical," skills are:
- Diagonal striding
- Double poling
- Kick double poling
- Uphill diagonal striding
- Herringbone

Freestyle skills for the more experienced skier are:
- Marathon skating
- Skating with poles
- Diagonal V (and variations)

The best advice we can give you is to warm up before you begin your workout. Cross-country skiing places extraordinary demands on your body. Additionally, you'll be dealing with cold, whose effects on anatomy and physiology have been well documented, and sometimes just being aware of them can help. For example, muscles start to fire less effectively when their temperature is dropped by as few as two degrees; aerobic capacity is decreased in direct proportion. So warming up muscles slowly before you hit the trail (we suggest active-isolated stretching) and wearing protective clothing might help give your muscles that edge against the cold they need. The cold can trick you into thinking that you're cooler than you are. When your skin is cold, it's easy to forget that your core temperature is rising to meet the physical requirements, and to warm your muscles as they fire. In fact, when you work hard, you sweat even when the temperature drops below zero! Dehydration doesn't take long to set in, which means that blood volumes diminish, and muscles struggle for oxygen that is delivered less and less with every stroke of your heart. Additionally, cells in your muscles—once plumped up with water—are drying out and shriveling. Microtearing and damage set in. Your heart rate increases to try and make up for the slack. Nothing works right. Fatigue sets in. You become less coordinated. And you lose the competition. Our simple message to you is *drink!* Additionally, beware of cold injuries such as windburn and frostbite. Protect exposed body parts with clothing specifically designed to keep you warm, wick perspiration out and block moisture from soaking in, maximize your aerodynamics, and "give" with every movement. And wear sunblock to screen out harmful rays reflected off the snow.

EQUIPMENT YOU'LL NEED

A watch
A bottle of water
Training inside:
    A ski-track machine
    Towel
Training outside:
    An identification card to put into your pocket
    Cell phone or walkie-talkie
    Skis
    Poles
    Boots

Bindings

Wax

Sunblock

Sunglasses

WHAT TO WEAR

When training inside, wear lightweight, comfortable clothing that will wick sweat away from your skin to keep you cool. Shorts and a shirt will do nicely. We suggest running shoes or aerobic dance shoes that provide support and protection to the balls of your feet. Wear socks.

When training outside, wear loose layers of warm clothing that you can add or shed easily. Layer 1: Next to your skin, wear long johns made from silk or polypropylene, which will wick sweat away from your body. Wear socks that will do the same. Make sure your socks fit snugly and are free from inside seams that will cause blisters on your feet. (Usually one pair of socks will do the trick, but some skiers prefer two.) Layer 2: Over the long johns, wear warm clothing like a wool turtleneck sweater with fitted cuffs to keep the snow off your wrists. Layer 3: A ski jacket and pants (or a combination suit) designed to weatherproof you. To protect your hands and keep them warm, wear gloves or mittens especially designed for skiing. Always wear a knit hat that you can pull down to cover your ears. Tuck a handkerchief or bandanna into your pocket.

BOREDOM BUSTERS

Training indoors:

Listen to music: Portable CD and tape players, and radios with lightweight headsets, are popular among our skiers. Just make sure that your choice of music is compatible with your planned workout: you want a steady tempo. Research has demonstrated that music can boost your workout without increasing your perception of effort.

Listen to books on tape: Raid your local library for books on tape—you could improve your mind and get through the classics while becoming fit. One of our clients listens only to biographies and autobiographies of athletes and coaches. He says it makes him feel that he's in the company of giants.

Watch TV: Training on the ski-track machine is one of the few workouts that allows your head to stay fairly steady. For this reason, you'll be able to focus on a television screen. Tune in your favorite program, turn up the sound just a little more than usual, and get to work. One of the advantages of television programs is that their usual length—one hour or thirty minutes—makes it easy for you to plan a workout around a program.

Training outdoors:

Recruit a partner: There's nothing like tracking next to a friend in the snow. Cross-country skiing is a sport of discovery and revelation. It's fun to share those exciting moments with someone who can appreciate them. Later, in the lodge, your friend can help you tell tall tales by the fireplace (although you should make a deal to embellish the heroics, but keep unflattering sprawls your little secret). Speaking of sprawls, another obvious advantage of skiing with a friend: there's safety in numbers. If you need help in the backcountry, you'll have a rescuer.

Be present: One of the skills most of us have lost in our hectic lives is the ability to just *be*. We're always reviewing things that have already happened or planning what's about to happen. Being in the moment is a particular challenge made easier by the silence of snow. Enjoy the experience of the skiing completely. And when you stop to rest, pay attention to your surroundings.

Take pictures: Tuck a small camera into your jacket pocket. Load it with 400 ASA film so you have a good chance of taking a successful photo with the white of the snow, the dark of the forest, and movement. Document your adventure. Looking for photo opportunities will focus your attention on the whole snowscape in new and interesting ways. Later, when summer comes, you'll have your photos to remind you that winter will indeed come again and soon you'll be back out on the trail.

Go on tour: If variety is the spice of life, then flavor your workout by changing your route. Go sight-seeing. One of the great joys of cross-country skiing is that you create your own trails. Just be sure you can find your way back to the lodge before dark.

TAKING IT TO THE GYM

Indoor ski-track machine

INJURY ALERT

Injuries, and they do occasionally occur, seem to center around trauma—accidents that happen when a skier using lightweight equipment reaches high speed, loses control, and falls or hits something. Studies also suggest that overuse or repetitive injuries of the shin, Achilles tendon, ankle, knee, and lower back are common. In fact, they might comprise 50 percent of all injuries that force a skier to lay off the sport for a significant period of healing. Experts agree that injury prevention is sometimes less a matter of physical conditioning and more a matter of learning how to select trails that are safe and free from potential hazards. Failing that, a cross-country skier should know how to fall without getting hurt. (Phil practices this all the time.)

TIPS FROM THE EXPERTS

A word about dehydration: it is deceptively easy to become dehydrated while skiing. Your body is losing water through exhalation and sweat, but you're hardly aware of it because you're in cold weather. And the telltale cottonmouth that serves as the first alert of dehydration is masked by the fact that your mouth is always dry when you breathe through it with exertion. The double whammy can mislead you. It's important that you drink before, during, and after skiing. Drink water or a sports beverage. An alcoholic hot toddy in the warming hut may warm your insides and quench your thirst, but it'll dehydrate you significantly, impede your reflexes, and cloud your judgment. Save it for later in the evening at the lodge.

COMING TO TERMS WITH THE TERMS WE USE IN YOUR SCHEDULE

Skate: This is a leisurely, conversational pace. You should be in the minimum range of your target heart rate.

Stride out: This is a quickened pace, but still conversational. You should be in the middle range of your target heart rate.

Sprint: This is race pace. You'll be exerting effort. You should be in the higher ranges of your target heart rate.

Surfaces: If we specify the topography (such as rolling hills or flat surfaces), do your best to follow our suggestions. If working out on specific surfaces isn't possible, any surface will do. If we haven't specified a surface, choose one you like.

DAY	1	Strength Work 2	3	Strength Work 4	5	Strength Work 6	7
WEEK 1 EASY	Make sure your equipment and clothing are in order.	Skate 15 min. on flat surface.	Skate 15 min. on flat surface.	Skate 15 min. Pick up the pace.	Rest.	Skate 5 min. at normal pace. Skate 15 min. Pick up the pace.	Skate 5 min. at normal pace. Skate 15 min. Pick up the pace.
2 MODERATE	Rest.	Skate 5 min. Stride out 5 min. (Easy does it!) Skate 5 min.	Skate 15 min. on flat surface.	Rest.	Skate 5 min. Stride out 5 min. (Easy does it!) Skate 5 min.	Rest.	Skate 5 min. at normal pace. Skate 15 min. Pick up the pace.
3 EASY							
4 HARD							
5 EASY							
6 HARD							

CROSS-COUNTRY SKIING BEGINNER *1. Awakening the Body*

CROSS-COUNTRY SKIING BEGINNER *2. Laying the Foundation*

DAY / WEEK	1	Strength Work 2	3	Strength Work 4	5	Strength Work 6	7
1 EASY	Rest.	Skate 20 min.	Skate 5 min. Skate/Stride out 20 min. (alternate skating and striding in 5-min. intervals). Skate 5 min.	Skate 20 min.	Rest.	Skate 20 min.	Skate 5 min. Skate/Stride out 10 min. (alternate skating and striding in 5-min. intervals). Skate 5 min.
2 MODERATE	Rest.	Skate 10 min. Stride out 20 min. Skate 10 min.	Skate 20 min. on flat surface.	Rest.	Skate 5 min. Skate/Stride out 10 min. (alternate skating and striding in 5-min. intervals). Skate 5 min.	Rest.	Skate 10 min. Stride out 5 min. Skate 10 min.
3 EASY	Rest.	Skate 25 min. on flat surface.	Rest.	Skate 25 min.	Rest.	Skate 5 min. Stride out 20 min.	Skate 5 min. Stride out 5 min. Skate 5 min. Stride out 5 min. Skate 5 min.
4 HARD	Rest.	Skate 5 min. Stride out 5 min. Skate 5 min. Stride out 5 min. Skate 5 min.	Stride out 25 min. Skate 5 min.	Skate 5 min. Stride out 5 min. Skate 5 min.	Rest.	Skate 20 min.	Skate 30 min.
5 EASY	Rest.	Skate 5 min. Stride out 10 min. Skate 5 min. Stride out 5 min. Skate 5 min.	Rest.	Rest.	Skate 5 min. Skate/Stride out 10 min. (alternate skating and striding in 1-min. intervals). Skate 10 min.	Rest.	Skate 5 min. Stride out 10 min. Skate 10 min.
6 HARD	Rest.	Skate 30 min.	Skate 5 min. Stride out 15 min. Skate 5 min.	Skate 10 min. Stride out 5 min. Skate 10 min.	Rest.	Skate 20 min.	Skate 5 min. Stride out 10 min. Skate 10 min.

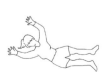

CROSS-COUNTRY SKIING BEGINNER 3. Building Endurance

DAY / WEEK	1	2 (Strength Work)	3	4 (Strength Work)	5	6 (Strength Work)	7
1 EASY	Rest.	Rolling hill work: Skate 5 min. Stride out 5 min. Skate 5 min. Skate 5 min.	Skate 5 min. Stride out 10 min. Skate 5 min.	Rest.	Rolling hill work: Skate 5 min. Stride out 10 min. Skate 5 min. Skate 5 min.	Rest.	Skate 5 min. Stride out 20 min. Skate 5 min.
2 MODERATE	Rest.	Rolling hill work: Skate 5 min. Stride out 10 min. Skate 5 min. Skate 5 min.	Stride out 5 min. Sprint 10 min. Stride out 5 min.	Skate 10 min. Stride out 10 min. Skate 10 min.	Rest.	Skate 5 min. Stride out 15 min. Skate 10 min.	Skate 5 min. Stride out 20 min. Skate 5 min.
3 EASY	Rest.	Rolling hill work: Skate 5 min. Stride out 10 min. Skate 5 min. Stride out 10 min. Skate 5 min.	Stride out 5 min. Sprint 15 min. Stride out 5 min.	Rest.	Rolling hill work: Skate 15 min. Stride out 15 min. Skate 10 min.	Rest.	Stride out 15 min. Sprint 20 min. Stride out 5 min.
4 HARD	Rest.	Rolling hill work: Skate 5 min. Stride out 20 min. Skate 5 min.	Stride out 5 min. Sprint 15 min. Stride out 5 min.	Rolling hill work: Skate 5 min. Stride out 5 min. Skate 5 min. Stride out 10 min. Skate 5 min.	Rest.	Skate 5 min. Stride out 20 min. Skate 5 min. Stride out 5 min. Skate 5 min.	Stride out 15 min. Sprint 25 min. Stride out 5 min.
5 EASY	Rest.	Rolling hill work: Skate 5 min. Stride out 15 min. Skate 5 min. Stride out 10 min. Skate 5 min.	Stride out 5 min. Sprint 20 min. Stride out 5 min.	Rest.	Rolling hill work: Skate 5 min. Stride out 10 min. Skate 5 min. Stride out 5 min. Skate 5 min.	Rest.	Stride out 25 min.
6 HARD	Rest.	Rolling hill work: Skate 5 min. Stride out 10 min. Skate 5 min. Stride out 15 min. Skate 5 min.	Skate 5 min. Stride out 25 min. Skate 5 min.	Skate 5 min. Stride out 5 min. Skate 5 min. Stride out 20 min. Skate 5 min.	Rest.	Stride out 5 min. Sprint 10 min. Stride out 5 min.	Stride out 30 min.

CROSS-COUNTRY SKIING BEGINNER *4. Achieving Mastery*

DAY	1	Strength Work 2	3	Strength Work 4	5	Strength Work 6	7
WEEK 1 EASY	Rest.	Rolling hill work: Stride out 5 min. Sprint 25 min. Stride out 5 min.	Stride out 5 min. Sprint 15 min. Stride out 5 min. Sprint 10 min. Stride out 5 min.	Rest.	Rolling hill work: Stride out 5 min. Sprint 5 min. Stride out 5 min. Repeat entire pattern.	Stride out 5 min. Sprint 20 min. Stride out 5 min.	Stride out 5 min. Sprint 25 min. Stride out 5 min.
2 MODERATE	Rest.	Rolling hill work: Stride out 5 min. Sprint 25 min. Stride out 5 min.	Stride out 5 min. Sprint 10 min. Stride out 5 min. Sprint 10 min. Stride out 5 min.	Rolling hill work: Stride out 5 min. Sprint 15 min. Stride out 5 min. Sprint 10 min. Stride out 5 min.	Rest.	Rolling hill work: Stride out 10 min. Sprint 15 min. Stride out 5 min.	Stride out 20 min. Sprint 10 min. Stride out 10 min.
3 EASY							
4 HARD							
5 EASY							
6 HARD							

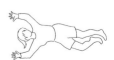

DAY	1	Strength Work 2	3	Strength Work 4	5	Strength Work 6	7
WEEK 1 EASY	Rest.	On flat surface: Stride out 5 min. Sprint 25 min. Stride out 5 min.	Stride out 5 min. Sprint 10 min. Stride out 5 min. Sprint 10 min. Stride out 5 min.	Rolling hill work: Stride out 5 min. Sprint 15 min. Stride out 5 min. Sprint 10 min. Stride out 5 min.	Rest.	Rolling hill work: Stride out 10 min. Sprint 15 min. Stride out 5 min.	Rolling hill work: Stride out 20 min. Sprint 10 min. Stride out 10 min.
2 MODERATE	Rest.	Rolling hill work: Stride out 10 min. Sprint 25 min. Stride out 10 min.	Stride out 5 min. Sprint 15 min. Stride out 5 min. Sprint 15 min. Stride out 5 min.	Rolling hill work: Stride out 10 min. For 30 min., alternate 1 min. sprinting with 1 min. striding. Stride out 5 min.	Rest.	Rolling hill work: Stride out 10 min. Sprint 20 min. Stride out 5 min.	Stride out 10 min. Sprint 20 min. Stride out 5 min.
3 EASY							
4 HARD							
5 EASY							
6 HARD							

CROSS-COUNTRY SKIING INTERMEDIATE   *6. Laying the Foundation*

DAY	1	2 (Strength Work)	3	4 (Strength Work)	5	6 (Strength Work)	7
WEEK 1 EASY	Rest.	Rolling hill work: Stride out 30 min.	Stride out 5 min. Sprint 15 min. Stride out 5 min. Sprint 15 min. Stride out 5 min.	Rolling hill work: Stride out 10 min. For 25 min., alternate 1 min. striding with 1 min. sprinting. Stride out 5 min.	Rest.	Rolling hill work: Stride out 10 min. Sprint 20 min. Stride out 5 min.	Rolling hill work: Stride out 10 min. Sprint 20 min. Stride out 5 min.
2 MODERATE	Rest.	Rolling hill work: Stride out 20 min. Sprint 10 min. Stride out 5 min.	On flat surface: Stride out 5 min. Sprint 20 min. Stride out 5 min. Sprint 10 min. Stride out 5 min.	Rolling hill work: Stride out 5 min. For 35 min., alternate 5 min. striding with 5 min. sprinting. Stride out 5 min.	Rest.	Rolling hill work: Stride out 5 min. Sprint 25 min. Stride out 5 min.	Rolling hill work: Stride out 10 min. Sprint 20 min. Stride out 5 min.
3 EASY	Rest.	Rolling hill work: Stride out 15 min. Sprint 10 min. Stride out 5 min.	Stride out 5 min. Sprint 15 min. Stride out 5 min. Sprint 10 min. Stride out 5 min.	Rolling hill work: Stride out 5 min. For 35 min., alternate 5 min. striding with 5 min. sprinting. Stride out 5 min.	Rest.	Rolling hill work: Stride out 35 min.	Rolling hill work: Stride out 10 min. Sprint 20 min. Stride out 5 min.
4 HARD	Rest.	Rolling hill work: Stride out 30 min. Sprint 15 min. Stride out 5 min.	Stride out 5 min. Sprint 20 min. Stride out 5 min. Sprint 10 min. Stride out 5 min.	Rolling hill work: Stride out 5 min. For 35 min., alternate 1 min. striding with 1 min. sprinting. Stride out 5 min.	Rest.	Rolling hill work: Stride out 25 min. Sprint 25 min. Stride out 5 min.	Rolling hill work: Stride out 10 min. Sprint 20 min. Stride out 5 min.
5 EASY	Rest.	Rolling hill work: Stride out 10 min. Sprint 10 min. Stride out 5 min.	Stride out 10 min. Sprint 10 min. Sprint 5 min. Stride out 5 min.	Rolling hill work: Stride out 5 min. For 35 min., alternate 5 min. striding with 5 min. sprinting. Stride out 5 min.	Rest.	Rolling hill work: Stride out 5 min. Sprint 25 min. Stride out 5 min.	Rolling hill work: Stride out 10 min. Sprint 20 min. Stride out 5 min. Sprint 5 min. Stride out 5 min.
6 HARD	Rest.	Rolling hill work: Stride out 10 min. Sprint 20 min. Stride out 5 min.	Stride out 10 min. Sprint 20 min. Stride out 5 min. Sprint 5 min. Stride out 5 min.	Rolling hill work: Stride out 5 min. For 35 min., alternate 5 min. striding with 5 min. sprinting. Stride out 5 min.	Rest.	Rolling hill work: Sprint 30 min. Stride out 5 min.	Rolling hill work: Stride out 10 min. Sprint 20 min. Stride out 5 min. Sprint 5 min. Stride out 5 min.

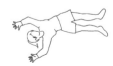

CROSS-COUNTRY SKIING INTERMEDIATE   *7. Building Endurance*

DAY / WEEK	1	Strength Work 2	3	Strength Work 4	5	Strength Work 6	7
1 EASY	Rest.	Rolling hill work: Sprint 15 min. Stride out 5 min.	Rolling hill work: Stride out 10 min. Sprint 10 min. Stride out 5 min.	Rolling hill work: Sprint 5 min. Stride out 2 min. Sprint 5 min. Stride out 5 min.	Rest.	Stride out 20 min. Sprint 5 min. Stride out 5 min.	Rolling hill work: Stride out 30 min.
2 MODERATE	Rest.	Rolling hill work: Sprint 15 min. Stride out 5 min.	Rolling hill work: Stride out 10 min. Sprint 10 min. Stride out 5 min.	Rolling hill work: Sprint 5 min. Stride out 2 min. Sprint 10 min. Stride out 5 min.	Rest.	Stride out 15 min. Sprint 10 min. Stride out 5 min.	Rolling hill work: Sprint 30 min.
3 EASY	Rest.	Rolling hill work: Sprint 15 min. Stride out 5 min.	Rolling hill work: Stride out 15 min. Sprint 10 min. Stride out 5 min.	Rolling hill work: Sprint 5 min. Stride out 2 min. Sprint 5 min. Stride out 5 min.	Rest.	Stride out 20 min. Sprint 5 min. Stride out 5 min.	Rolling hill work: Sprint 30 min.
4 HARD	Rest.	Rolling hill work: Sprint 20 min. Stride out 5 min.	Rolling hill work: Stride out 15 min. Sprint 10 min. Stride out 5 min.	Rolling hill work: Sprint 5 min. Stride out 2 min. Sprint 7 min. Stride out 5 min.	Rest.	Stride out 20 min. Sprint 10 min. Stride out 5 min.	Rolling hill work: Sprint 30 min.
5 EASY	Rest.	Rolling hill work: Sprint 20 min. Stride out 5 min.	Rolling hill work: Stride out 15 min. Sprint 10 min. Stride out 5 min.	Rolling hill work: Sprint 5 min. Stride out 2 min. Sprint 7 min. Stride out 5 min.	Rest.	Stride out 20 min. Sprint 10 min. Stride out 5 min.	Rolling hill work: Sprint 35 min.
6 HARD	Rest.	Rolling hill work: Sprint 25 min. Stride out 5 min.	Rest.	Rolling hill work: Sprint 10 min. Stride out 2 min. Sprint 10 min. Stride out 5 min.	Rest.	Stride out 30 min.	Rolling hill work: Sprint 35 min.

DAY	1	Strength Work 2	3	Strength Work 4	5	Strength Work 6	7
WEEK 1 EASY	Rest.	Rolling hill work: Sprint 35 min.	Rolling hill work: Stride out 5 min. Sprint 5 min. Stride out 5 min. Sprint 7 min. Stride out 5 min.	Rolling hill work: Stride out 10 min. Sprint 10 min. Stride out 10 min.	Rest.	Stride out 15 min. Sprint 10 min. Stride out 2 min.	Rolling hill work: Sprint 35 min. Stride out 5 min.
2 MODERATE	Rest.	Rolling hill work: Sprint 35 min.	Rolling hill work: Stride out 5 min. Sprint 10 min. Stride out 5 min. Sprint 7 min. Stride out 5 min.	Rolling hill work: Sprint 25 min. Stride out 5 min.	Rest.	Stride out 20 min. Sprint 10 min. Stride out 2 min.	Rolling hill work: Sprint 35 min. Stride out 5 min.
3 EASY	Rest.	Rolling hill work: Sprint 35 min.	Rest.	Rolling hill work: Sprint 20 min. Stride out 5 min.	Rest.	Stride out 15 min. Sprint 10 min. Stride out 2 min.	Rolling hill work: Sprint 35 min. Stride out 5 min.
4 HARD	Rest.	Rolling hill work: Sprint 35 min.	Rolling hill work: Sprint 20 min. Stride out 5 min.	Rolling hill work: Sprint 25 min. Stride out 5 min.	Rest.	Stride out 10 min. Sprint 20 min. Stride out 2 min.	Rolling hill work: Sprint 35 min. Stride out 5 min.
5 EASY							
6 HARD							

CROSS-COUNTRY SKIING ADVANCED   *9. Awakening the Body*

DAY	1	Strength Work 2	3	Strength Work 4	5	Strength Work 6	7
WEEK 1 EASY	Rest.	Rolling hill work: Sprint 25 min. Stride out 5 min.	Stride out 10 min. Sprint 20 min. Stride out 5 min.	Stride out 5 min. Sprint 15 min. Stride out 10 min.	Rest.	Stride out 20 min. Sprint 20 min. Stride out 5 min.	Rolling hill work: Sprint 45 min. Stride out 5 min.
2 MODERATE	Rest.	Rolling hill work: Sprint 30 min. Stride out 5 min.	Rest.	Rolling hill work: Sprint 25 min. Stride out 5 min.	Rest.	Stride out 40 min.	Rolling hill work: Sprint 45 min. Stride out 5 min.
3 EASY							
4 HARD							
5 EASY							
6 HARD							

CROSS-COUNTRY SKIING ADVANCED *10. Laying the Foundation*

DAY	1	Strength Work 2	3	Strength Work 4	5	Strength Work 6	7
WEEK 1 EASY	Rest.	Rolling hill work: Sprint 35 min. Stride out 5 min.	Rolling hill work: Stride out 5 min. Sprint 30 min. Stride out 5 min.	Stride out 15 min. Sprint 10 min. Stride out 5 min.	Rest.	Stride out 20 min. Sprint 20 min.	Rolling hill work: Sprint 40 min. Stride out 5 min.
2 MODERATE	Rest.	Rolling hill work: Sprint 35 min. Stride out 5 min.	Rolling hill work: Stride out 5 min. Sprint 40 min. Stride out 5 min.	Stride out 20 min. Sprint 10 min. Stride out 5 min.	Rest.	Stride out 40 min.	Rolling hill work: Sprint 40 min. Stride out 5 min.
3 EASY	Rest.	Rolling hill work: Sprint 35 min. Stride out 5 min.	Rest.	Stride out 20 min. Sprint 10 min. Stride out 5 min.	Rest.	Stride out 20 min. Sprint 30 min.	Rolling hill work: Sprint 40 min. Stride out 5 min.
4 HARD	Rest.	Rolling hill work: Sprint 35 min. Stride out 5 min.	Rolling hill work: Stride out 5 min. Sprint 40 min. Stride out 5 min.	Stride out 25 min. Sprint 15 min. Stride out 5 min.	Rest.	Stride out 10 min. Sprint 20 min.	Rolling hill work: Sprint 40 min. Stride out 5 min.
5 EASY	Rest.	Rolling hill work: Sprint 35 min. Stride out 5 min.	Game Day.	Stride out 20 min. Sprint 20 min.	Rest.	Stride out 20 min. Sprint 20 min.	Rolling hill work: Sprint 40 min. Stride out 5 min.
6 HARD	Rest.	Rolling hill work: Sprint 35 min. Stride out 5 min.	Game Day.	Stride out 15 min. Sprint 30 min.	Rest.	Stride out 20 min. Sprint 20 min.	Rolling hill work: Sprint 40 min. Stride out 5 min.

DAY	1	Strength Work 2	3	Strength Work 4	5	Strength Work 6	7
WEEK 1 EASY	Rest.	Sprint 35 min. Keep a steady pace.	Game Day.	Stride out 10 min. Sprint 30 min. Stride out 5 min.	Rest.	Stride out 20 min. Sprint 20 min.	Sprint 45 min. Keep a steady pace.
2 MODERATE	Rest.	Sprint 40 min. Keep a steady pace.	Game Day.	Stride out 5 min. Sprint 40 min. Stride out 5 min.	Rest.	Stride out 20 min. Sprint 20 min.	Sprint 45 min. Keep a steady pace.
3 EASY	Rest.	Sprint 35 min. Keep a steady pace.	Game Day.	Sprint 45 min. Stride out 5 min.	Rest.	Stride out 20 min. Sprint 20 min.	Sprint 45 min. Keep a steady pace.
4 HARD	Rest.	Sprint 45 min. Keep a steady pace.	Game Day.	Sprint 45 min. Stride out 5 min.	Rest.	Stride out 20 min. Sprint 20 min.	Sprint 50 min. Keep a steady pace.
5 EASY	Rest.	Stride out 5 min. Sprint 15 min. Stride out 5 min. Sprint 15 min. Stride out 5 min.	Sprint 40 min. Keep a steady pace.	Game Day.	Rest.	Sprint 30 min. Keep a steady pace.	Stride out 45 min. Keep a steady pace.
6 HARD	Rest.	Stride out 5 min. Sprint 20 min. Stride out 5 min. Sprint 20 min. Stride out 5 min.	Sprint 45 min. Keep a steady pace.	Game Day.	Rest.	Sprint 30 min. Keep a steady pace.	Sprint 50 min. Keep a steady pace.

CROSS-COUNTRY SKIING ADVANCED *11. Building Endurance*

CROSS-COUNTRY SKIING ADVANCED   12. Achieving Mastery

DAY	1	Strength Work 2	3	Strength Work 4	5	Strength Work 6	7
WEEK 1 EASY	Rest.	Stride out 5 min. Sprint 20 min. Stride out 5 min. Sprint 10 min. Stride out 5 min.	Sprint 40 min.	Game Day.	Rest.	Sprint 30 min.	Sprint 45 min.
2 MODERATE	Rest.	Stride out 5 min. Sprint 25 min. Stride out 5 min. Sprint 5 min. Stride out 5 min.	Sprint 50 min.	Game Day.	Rest.	Sprint 30 min.	Sprint 55 min.
3 EASY	Rest.	Stride out 5 min. Sprint 35 min. Stride out 10 min.	Sprint 30 min.	Game Day.	Rest.	Sprint 30 min.	Sprint 40 min.
4 HARD	Rest.	Sprint 35 min.	Sprint 40 min.	Sprint 30 min.	Rest.	Sprint 30 min.	Sprint 60 min.
5 EASY							
6 HARD							

CYCLING

See art, pages 165–183.

TECHNIQUE AND FORM

We assume that you already know how to ride. Needless to say, you can't learn to ride a bike from a book, including ours. If you don't know how to ride, contact a local bike shop or cycling club for the names of cyclists who are willing to instruct you.

Cycling started out as basic transportation and remains so for many people around the world, but for a select few who love the complex relationship and mystical partnership of human body and machine, cycling's been elevated to art. The rest of us just enjoy it. It's a sport for nearly everyone. And it's a great workout.

In cycling, leg muscles are primary performers. When depressing the pedal, you use hip and knee extensors (quads) and ankle flexors (tibialis anterior). In raising the pedal, you use your hip and knee flexors (hamstrings) and ankle extensors (gastrocnemius muscles). You use these muscles consistently, particularly with the use of toe clips that lock the feet into position. Your arm extensors help you steer, and support some of the weight of your trunk as you lean into the handlebars in that signature aerodynamic position. But your trunk isn't just along for the ride; your back and abdominals serve as your foundation for stability—transmitting the support work of your arms to your legs. And your upper back and neck are holding your head up. It helps to see where you're going. Additionally, as you pump, you're getting a no-impact aerobic workout (hopefully *no*-impact).

As you ride, give your body a break by sitting upright from time to time to take the pressure off your back and neck. Stand up in the pedals and get the pressure off your butt. Remove your hands from the handlegrips one at a time, shake them out, and flex your fingers to get blood flowing.

EQUIPMENT YOU'LL NEED

A watch
A bottle of water clipped to the frame of your bike
An identification card to put into your pocket
Cell phone (perhaps in a bike pack)
Repair kit and extra tire tube

Pump

Lock and key

Bicycle: Experts advise to shop for a bike in a store that specializes in bikes. It makes sense. Not only is their selection more refined than a general retailer, but these stores tend to be staffed by cycling enthusiasts who are as knowledgeable as they are passionate. Additionally, most bike shops have a repair department. Having an up-close and personal relationship with a repair department comes in handy when something breaks or you want to add or modify equipment on your bike. The kind of bike will vary with your wants, needs, and bank account balance, but generally adult bikes fall into three categories: mountain bikes, road bikes, and hybrid bikes (a cross between mountain and road).

Mountain bike: Handles trails, off-road, on-road, commuting, and touring. Rider sits upright. Tires are wide. Controls are easy to reach. Low maintenance. Few gears.

Road bike: Handles well on-road and in commuting, and racing. Dropped handlebars put rider in aerodynamic posture. Tires are narrow and easily punctured. Controls easy to reach.

Hybrid bike: Heavier and slower than the road bike, lighter and faster than the mountain bike. Handles trails, off-road, on-road, and commuting. Rider sits upright. Tires are wide.

Do your homework before you walk into a bike shop. You can research possible choices by browsing cycling magazines and websites, and by talking to other cyclists. Make sure the bike frame fits your body well and that the seat, handlebars, and pedals are adjusted to your measurements. Make sure the seat is comfortable and will remain so mile after mile after mile. Insist that you be allowed to road test a bike before you purchase it. Stick to your budget.

WHAT TO WEAR

In cycling, you can wear almost anything, but we recommend clothing made for cycling.

Shorts: Bike shorts fit snugly from the waist to the midthigh, and are made mostly of nylon or Lycra. The secret pleasure of bike shorts is that they're padded to help cushion delicate anatomical parts that make direct contact with an unyielding saddle. The longer the duration of your ride, the more you'll appreciate the padding. Men's and women's shorts are fitted and padded specifically for the gender, so pay close attention to the tag when you're trying them on.

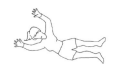

Jerseys: Of course we could tell you that any old T-shirt will do, but the truth is that a cycling jersey is a better choice. It's lightweight and has sleeves that protect the shoulders from abrasion in a tumble. Another difference between a cycling jersey and "any old T-shirt" is that the jersey has pockets stitched into the back, where you can slip a water bottle and a snack for a long ride. Choose a jersey made of a fabric that wicks sweat away from your body and helps keep you cool.

Shoes: You can ride with running shoes, but a cycling shoe is less flexible and designed to fit the pedal and keep your foot from fatiguing and slipping.

Gloves: Cycling gloves are padded in the palms to absorb some of the pressure from your leaning on the handlegrips. Additionally, they keep your hands warm in the wind and protect your hands in the event you take a tumble.

Sunglasses: Wear impact-resistant sunglasses to protect your eyes from UVA, the glare of the road, and airborne debris that might otherwise find its way into your eye as you rocket along.

Helmet: This is non-negotiable. Wear one. Every time.

Socks: Socks are optional, but most cyclists appreciate them. They add a layer of protection between your foot and the inside of the shoe. Look for a smooth, snug fit that's free from wrinkles and inside seams. Because even the best socks are an inexpensive investment, go first-class. Purchase athletes' socks that are engineered to "wick" moisture, or absorb sweat away from your foot, and provide you with a dryer shoe interior, which will help prevent blistering, skin irritations, and odor. Treat yourself to a clean pair of socks with every workout.

BOREDOM BUSTERS

Listen to music: Portable CD and tape players, and radios with lightweight headsets, are popular among cyclists. Just make sure that your choice of music is compatible with your planned workout. If you're riding in the company of other people, be sure you're using a headset that affords you complete privacy. In other words, do everything possible to keep from imposing (or inflicting) your choice of music—and its accompanying rhythms—on others. Before you use a headset, make sure it's legal. When using a headset, leave one ear totally free so that you can hear what's going on around you and stay alert to your environment.

Recruit a partner: There's safety in numbers. There's also motivation. You and a friend can work together to keep your training schedules on track. Better yet, join a club or a cycling group where you can work out with other cyclists.

Sign up for an event: Nothing motivates a cyclist like an upcoming competition or a benefit ride. Targeting a specific goal on a specific date puts focus and excitement into even the most anemic program. And there's nothing like a souvenir T-shirt for spicing up your wardrobe like a veteran. There are lots of cycling events for charities.

Use your bike for transportation: While it's fun to work out on your bike or ride recreationally, it's a nice change of pace to use the bike for basic transportation. If you can, run errands or visit friends on your bike.

Play tourist: Use your bike to explore new places. If you have to, rack your bike onto the car and take it somewhere you've never been. Pack a picnic, gather a few friends, and head off on an adventure. If you're not sure where to go, check with the local, county, and state parks services that serve your area. You'll find a wealth of bike path information, including greenways that are bicycle-friendly. For ideas, jump onto the Internet; bike clubs all over the country post their best, most interesting routes and maps on their websites.

TAKING IT TO THE GYM

Stationary bike
Recumbent bike
Stationary trainer

INJURY ALERT

Because cycling is a repetitive sport, overuse injuries are the most common. Cyclists are susceptible to nerve compression of the hand (ulnar nerve) and forearm (radial distal nerve). Contracted muscles tighten up and put the nerves in a strangle hold, causing pain, numbness, fatigue, weakness, and irritation. We also see some nerve compression in the foot. The causes are tight shoes, too short a distance between the seat and the pedals, putting too much force on the pedal for extended periods of time, and weak muscles of the lower leg. Flexibility training will probably get you out of nerve compression, but it may take some time before you are 100 percent. We see inflammation of the tendons at their attachments at the hip, knee, and ankle, and overly tight quadriceps compressing the kneecap against the joint (major discomfort), pressure on the nerves of the cervical spine at the back of the neck from hyperextending and fatiguing the neck in holding the head up, low back pain, and pain deep in the buttocks (sciatica). Flexibility and strength will prevent all these problems.

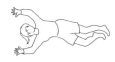

A couple of words about crashing: it happens. This is why we caution cyclists to be on guard at all times, to ride within their physical capabilities, and to wear a helmet. Remember the rules of the road: ride with automobile traffic, not against it.

TIPS FROM THE EXPERTS

In truth, cycling can be an invaluable cardiovascular component in a comprehensive fitness program. In fact, it can provide the stellar benefits of running without the impact on feet, legs, and hips. You'll get the best out of cycling if you learn how to ride properly and have the right bike. Work up slowly in intensity, distance, and duration.

A final note: please remember to hydrate when you ride. Cyclists sometimes forget how much they are sweating and that they need to replenish fluids. As a cyclist rockets along the road, air passes over his body, evaporating the sweat and cooling his skin. He's riding in a constant breeze that automatically adjusts itself to his speed. He rides slowly and experiences a gentle breeze; he rides fast and experiences a gale force wind. The problem is that the cyclist may be deceived into thinking that cool and comfortable skin equals a cool and comfortable core temperature. Wrong. Heat problems set in when dehydration lowers the circulating volume of blood and the core temperature starts to rise. Problems manifest themselves in symptoms that include fatigue, lack of coordination, muscle pain and cramping, headache, light-headedness, confusion, disorientation, and fainting. Under extreme circumstances, death can occur. If you feel thirsty, you're already on your way to trouble. Drink early—before thirst sets in—and often. Experts say that water is perfect for short workouts, but a commercial sport fluid-replacement drink is preferable for workouts of more than ninety minutes in duration. With either choice, *cold* is best. We want you to play it cool. Drink. Get a water bottle attachment for your bike frame and fill it before you start your workout.

COMING TO TERMS WITH THE TERMS WE USE IN YOUR SCHEDULE

Easy effort: This is a leisurely, conversational pace. You should be in the minimum range of your target heart rate.

Moderate effort: This is a quickened pace, but still conversational. You should be in the middle range of your target heart rate.

Hard effort: This is race pace. You'll be exerting effort. You should be in the higher ranges of your target heart rate.

Surfaces: If we specify the topography (such as rolling hills or flat surfaces), do your best to follow our suggestions. If working out on specific surfaces isn't possible, any surface will do. If we haven't specified a surface, choose one you like.

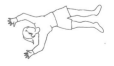

CYCLING BEGINNER 1. Awakening the Body

DAY	1	2	3	4	5	6	7
		Strength Work		Strength Work		Strength Work	
WEEK 1 EASY	Make sure your bike and clothing are in order.	Cycle 15 min. Easy effort.	Cycle 15 min. Easy effort.	Cycle 15 min. Easy effort.	Rest.	Cycle 10 min. Easy effort. 5 min. Moderate effort.	Cycle 15 min. Easy effort. 5 min. Moderate effort.
2 MODERATE	Rest.	Cycle 10 min. Easy effort. 5 min. Moderate effort.	Cycle 15 min. Easy effort. 5 min. Moderate effort.	Rest.	Cycle 15 min. Easy effort. 5 min. Moderate effort.	Rest.	Cycle 15 min. Easy effort. 5 min. Moderate effort.
3 EASY							
4 HARD							
5 EASY							
6 HARD							

CYCLING BEGINNER 2. Laying the Foundation

DAY	1	Strength Work 2	3	Strength Work 4	5	Strength Work 6	7
WEEK 1 EASY	Rest.	Cycle 15 min. Easy effort. 5 min. Moderate effort.	Rest.	Cycle 25 min. Easy effort.	Rest.	Cycle 25 min. Easy effort.	Cycle 20 min. Easy effort. 5 min. Moderate effort.
2 MODERATE	Rest.	Cycle 10 min. Easy effort. 10 min. Moderate effort.	Cycle 15 min. Easy effort. 10 min. Moderate effort.	Rest.	Cycle 15 min. Easy effort. 10 min. Moderate effort.	Rest.	Cycle 20 min. Easy effort. 10 min. Moderate effort.
3 EASY	Rest.	Cycle 20 min. Easy effort. 5 min. Moderate effort.	Rest.	Cycle 20 min. Easy effort. 5 min. Moderate effort.	Rest.	Cycle 20 min. Easy effort.	Cycle 25 min. Easy effort. 5 min. Moderate effort.
4 HARD	Rest.	Cycle 20 min. Easy effort. 10 min. Moderate effort.	Cycle 20 min. Easy effort. 5 min. Moderate effort.	Cycle 20 min. Easy effort. 10 min. Moderate effort.	Rest.	Cycle 20 min. Easy effort. 10 min. Moderate effort.	Rolling hill work: Cycle 15 min. Easy effort. 5 min. Moderate effort.
5 EASY	Rest.	Cycle 20 min. Easy effort. 5 min. Moderate effort.	Rest.	Rest.	Rolling hill work: Cycle 15 min. Easy effort. 5 min. Moderate effort.	Rest.	Cycle 25 min. Easy effort. 10 min. Moderate effort.
6 HARD	Rest.	Rolling hill work: Cycle 20 min. Easy effort. 10 min. Moderate effort.	Cycle 20 min. Easy effort. 5 min. Moderate effort.	Rolling hill work: Cycle 20 min. Easy effort. 10 min. Moderate effort.	Rest.	Cycle 30 min. Easy effort. 10 min. Moderate effort.	Rolling hill work: Cycle 20 min. Easy effort. 15 min. Moderate effort.

DAY	1	Strength Work 2	3	Strength Work 4	5	Strength Work 6	7
WEEK 1 EASY	Rest.	Rolling hill work: Cycle 20 min. Easy effort. 10 min. Moderate effort.	Cycle 15 min. Easy effort. 5 min. Moderate effort.	Rest.	Cycle 20 min. Easy effort. 10 min. Moderate effort.	Rest.	Rolling hill work: Cycle 15 min. Easy effort. 5 min. Moderate effort.
2 MODERATE	Rest.	Rolling hill work: Cycle 20 min. Easy effort. 15 min. Moderate effort.	Cycle 15 min. Easy effort. 10 min. Moderate effort.	Rolling hill work: Cycle 15 min. Easy effort. 10 min. Moderate effort.	Rest.	Cycle 15 min. Easy effort. 5 min. Moderate effort.	Rolling hill work: Cycle 15 min. Easy effort. 10 min. Moderate effort.
3 EASY	Rest.	Rolling hill work: Cycle 20 min. Easy effort. 10 min. Moderate effort.	Cycle 15 min. Easy effort. 5 min. Moderate effort.	Rest.	Rolling hill work: Cycle 20 min. Easy effort. 10 min. Moderate effort.	Rest.	Cycle 20 min. Moderate effort. 10 min. Hard effort.
4 HARD	Rest.	Rolling hill work: Cycle 25 min. Easy effort. 10 min. Moderate effort.	Cycle 15 min. Easy effort. 15 min. Moderate effort.	Rolling hill work: Cycle 25 min. Easy effort. 15 min. Moderate effort.	Rest.	Cycle 20 min. Moderate effort. 10 min. Hard effort.	Cycle 20 min. Moderate effort. 15 min. Hard effort.
5 EASY	Rest.	Rolling hill work: Cycle 20 min. Easy effort. 10 min. Moderate effort.	Rolling hill work: Cycle 15 min. Easy effort. 10 min. Moderate effort.	Rest.	Rolling hill work: Cycle 20 min. Easy effort. 10 min. Moderate effort.	Rest.	Cycle 25 min. Moderate effort.
6 HARD	Rest.	Rolling hill work: Cycle 15 min. Moderate effort. 10 min. Hard effort.	Rolling hill work: Cycle 15 min. Moderate effort. 15 min. Hard effort.	Cycle 20 min. Moderate effort. 20 min. Hard effort.	Rest.	Cycle 20 min. Moderate effort. 20 min. Hard effort.	Cycle 30 min. Moderate effort.

CYCLING BEGINNER   *3. Building Endurance*

DAY	1	Strength Work 2	3	Strength Work 4	5	Strength Work 6	7
WEEK 1 EASY	Rest.	Rolling hill work: Cycle 15 min. Moderate effort. 10 min. Hard effort.	Rolling hill work: Cycle 15 min. Moderate effort. 15 min. Hard effort.	Rest.	Rolling hill work: Cycle 15 min. Moderate effort. 15 min. Hard effort.	Rolling hill work: Cycle 20 min. Moderate effort. 15 min. Hard effort.	Cycle 10 min. Moderate effort. 20 min. Hard effort.
2 MODERATE	Rest.	Rolling hill work: Cycle 15 min. Moderate effort. 15 min. Hard effort.	Rolling hill work: Cycle 20 min. Moderate effort. 15 min. Hard effort.	Rolling hill work: Cycle 15 min. Moderate effort. 15 min. Hard effort.	Rest.	Rolling hill work: Cycle 15 min. Moderate effort. 15 min. Hard effort.	Cycle 15 min. Moderate effort. 25 min. Hard effort.
3 EASY							
4 HARD							
5 EASY							
6 HARD							

CYCLING BEGINNER *4. Achieving Mastery*

10. The Ten Best Cardio-Fit Activities and Training Schedules   **211**

CYCLING INTERMEDIATE   5. Awakening the Body

DAY	1	Strength Work 2	3	Strength Work 4	5	Strength Work 6	7
WEEK 1 EASY	Rest.	Rolling hill work: Cycle 10 min. Moderate effort. 15 min. Hard effort.	Cycle 15 min. Moderate effort. 15 min. Hard effort.	Rolling hill work: Cycle 10 min. Moderate effort. 15 min. Hard effort.	Rest.	Rolling hill work: Cycle 15 min. Moderate effort. 15 min. Hard effort.	Rolling hill work: Cycle 20 min. Moderate effort. 10 min. Hard effort.
2 MODERATE	Rest.	Rolling hill work: Cycle 15 min. Moderate effort. 15 min. Hard effort.	Cycle 20 min. Moderate effort. 15 min. Hard effort.	Rolling hill work: Cycle 20 min. Moderate effort. 15 min. Hard effort.	Rest.	Rolling hill work: Cycle 20 min. Moderate effort. 15 min. Hard effort.	Rolling hill work: Cycle 15 min. Moderate effort. 20 min. Hard effort.
3 EASY							
4 HARD							
5 EASY							
6 HARD							

DAY	1	Strength Work 2	3	Strength Work 4	5	Strength Work 6	7
WEEK 1 EASY	Rest.	Rolling hill work: Cycle 15 min. Moderate effort. 15 min. Hard effort.	Cycle 15 min. Moderate effort. 15 min. Hard effort.	Rolling hill work: Cycle 15 min. Moderate effort. 15 min. Hard effort.	Rest.	Rolling hill work: Cycle 10 min. Moderate effort. 10 min. Hard effort.	Rolling hill work: Cycle 15 min. Moderate effort. 15 min. Hard effort.
2 MODERATE	Rest.	Rolling hill work: Cycle 20 min. Moderate effort. 20 min. Hard effort.	Cycle 20 min. Moderate effort. 15 min. Hard effort.	Rolling hill work: Cycle 15 min. Moderate effort. 15 min. Hard effort.	Rest.	Rolling hill work: Cycle 15 min. Moderate effort. 10 min. Hard effort.	Rolling hill work: Cycle 20 min. Moderate effort. 15 min. Hard effort.
3 EASY	Rest.	Rolling hill work: Cycle 15 min. Moderate effort. 15 min. Hard effort.	Rolling hill work: Cycle 15 min. Moderate effort. 15 min. Hard effort.	Rolling hill work: Cycle 15 min. Moderate effort. 10 min. Hard effort.	Rest.	Rolling hill work: Cycle 25 min. Moderate effort.	Rolling hill work: Cycle 15 min. Moderate effort. 15 min. Hard effort.
4 HARD	Rest.	Rolling hill work: Cycle 20 min. Moderate effort. 20 min. Hard effort.	Cycle 20 min. Moderate effort. 20 min. Hard effort.	Rolling hill work: Cycle 20 min. Moderate effort. 15 min. Hard effort.	Rest.	Rolling hill work: Cycle 20 min. Moderate effort. 20 min. Hard effort.	Rolling hill work: Cycle 25 min. Moderate effort. 15 min. Hard effort.
5 EASY	Rest.	Rolling hill work: Cycle 20 min. Moderate effort. 15 min. Hard effort.	Cycle 15 min. Moderate effort. 15 min. Hard effort.	Rolling hill work: Cycle 20 min. Moderate effort. 10 min. Hard effort.	Rest.	Rolling hill work: Cycle 20 min. Moderate effort. 15 min. Hard effort.	Rolling hill work: Cycle 20 min. Moderate effort. 15 min. Hard effort.
6 HARD	Rest.	Rolling hill work: Cycle 20 min. Moderate effort. 20 min. Hard effort.	Cycle 25 min. Moderate effort. 20 min. Hard effort.	Rolling hill work: Cycle 20 min. Moderate effort. 20 min. Hard effort.	Rest.	Rolling hill work: Cycle 20 min. Moderate effort. 15 min. Hard effort.	Rolling hill work: Cycle 25 min. Moderate effort. 20 min. Hard effort.

CYCLING INTERMEDIATE   *6. Laying the Foundation*

DAY	1	Strength Work 2	3	Strength Work 4	5	Strength Work 6	7
WEEK 1 EASY	Rest.	Rolling hill work: Cycle 20 min. Moderate effort. 15 min. Hard effort.	Rolling hill work: Cycle 15 min. Moderate effort. 15 min. Hard effort.	Rolling hill work: Cycle 20 min. Moderate effort. 15 min. Hard effort.	Rest.	Cycle 20 min. Moderate effort. 25 min. Hard effort.	Rolling hill work: Cycle 25 min. Moderate effort.
2 MODERATE	Rest.	Rolling hill work: Cycle 20 min. Moderate effort. 20 min. Hard effort.	Rolling hill work: Cycle 20 min. Moderate effort. 15 min. Hard effort.	Rolling hill work: Cycle 20 min. Moderate effort. 20 min. Hard effort.	Rest.	Cycle 20 min. Moderate effort. 20 min. Hard effort.	Rolling hill work: Cycle 35 min. Moderate effort.
3 EASY	Rest.	Rolling hill work: Cycle 20 min. Moderate effort. 15 min. Hard effort.	Rolling hill work: Cycle 15 min. Moderate effort. 15 min. Hard effort.	Rolling hill work: Cycle 20 min. Moderate effort. 15 min. Hard effort.	Rest.	Cycle 20 min. Moderate effort. 25 min. Hard effort.	Rolling hill work: Cycle 30 min. Moderate effort.
4 HARD	Rest.	Rolling hill work: Cycle 25 min. Moderate effort. 20 min. Hard effort.	Rolling hill work: Cycle 20 min. Moderate effort. 15 min. Hard effort.	Rolling hill work: Cycle 25 min. Moderate effort. 20 min. Hard effort.	Rest.	Cycle 30 min. Moderate effort. 20 min. Hard effort.	Rolling hill work: Cycle 40 min. Moderate effort.
5 EASY	Rest.	Rolling hill work: Cycle 20 min. Moderate effort. 15 min. Hard effort.	Rolling hill work: Cycle 20 min. Moderate effort. 25 min. Hard effort.	Rolling hill work: Cycle 20 min. Moderate effort. 15 min. Hard effort.	Rest.	Cycle 20 min. Moderate effort. 25 min. Hard effort.	Rolling hill work: Cycle 35 min. Moderate effort.
6 HARD	Rest.	Rolling hill work: Cycle 25 min. Moderate effort. 25 min. Hard effort.	Rest.	Rolling hill work: Cycle 25 min. Moderate effort. 25 min. Hard effort.	Rest.	Cycle 50 min. Moderate effort.	Rolling hill work: Cycle 40 min. Moderate effort.

CYCLING INTERMEDIATE   *7. Building Endurance*

DAY	1	Strength Work 2	3	Strength Work 4	5	Strength Work 6	7
WEEK 1 EASY	Rest.	Rolling hill work: Cycle 25 min. Moderate effort. 25 min. Hard effort.	Rolling hill work: Cycle 20 min. Moderate effort. 20 min. Hard effort.	Rolling hill work: Cycle 25 min. Moderate effort. 25 min. Hard effort.	Rest.	Cycle 30 min. Moderate effort. 20 min. Hard effort.	Rolling hill work: Cycle 30 min. Moderate effort. 20 min. Hard effort.
2 MODERATE	Rest.	Rolling hill work: Cycle 30 min. Moderate effort. 25 min. Hard effort.	Rolling hill work: Cycle 35 min. Moderate effort. 25 min. Hard effort.	Rolling hill work: Cycle 30 min. Moderate effort. 25 min. Hard effort.	Rest.	Cycle 35 min. Moderate effort. 25 min. Hard effort.	Rolling hill work: Cycle 35 min. Moderate effort. 25 min. Hard effort.
3 EASY	Rest.	Rolling hill work: Cycle 25 min. Moderate effort. 25 min. Hard effort.	Rest.	Rolling hill work: Cycle 30 min. Moderate effort. 25 min. Hard effort.	Rest.	Cycle 25 min. Moderate effort. 25 min. Hard effort.	Rolling hill work: Cycle 25 min. Moderate effort. 25 min. Hard effort.
4 HARD	Rest.	Rolling hill work: Cycle 30 min. Moderate effort. 30 min. Hard effort.	Rolling hill work: Cycle 35 min. Moderate effort. 30 min. Hard effort.	Rolling hill work: Cycle 30 min. Moderate effort. 30 min. Hard effort.	Rest.	Cycle 40 min. Moderate effort. 25 min. Hard effort.	Rolling hill work: Cycle 40 min. Moderate effort. 25 min. Hard effort.
5 EASY							
6 HARD							

CYCLING INTERMEDIATE   *8. Achieving Mastery*

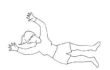

CYCLING ADVANCED   9. *Awakening the Body*

DAY / WEEK	1	Strength Work 2	3	Strength Work 4	5	Strength Work 6	7
WEEK 1 EASY	Rest.	Rolling hill work: Cycle 25 min. Moderate effort. 25 min. Hard effort.	Cycle 40 min. Moderate effort.	Cycle 25 min. Moderate effort. 25 min. Hard effort.	Rest.	Cycle 45 min. Moderate effort.	Rolling hill work: Cycle 25 min. Moderate effort. 25 min. Hard effort.
2 MODERATE	Rest.	Rolling hill work: Cycle 35 min. Moderate effort. 25 min. Hard effort.	Rest.	Rolling hill work: Cycle 40 min. Moderate effort. 25 min. Hard effort.	Rest.	Cycle 50 min. Moderate effort.	Rolling hill work: Cycle 30 min. Moderate effort. 25 min. Hard effort.
3 EASY							
4 HARD							
5 EASY							
6 HARD							

DAY	1	2 Strength Work	3	4 Strength Work	5	6 Strength Work	7
WEEK 1 EASY	Rest.	Rolling hill work: Cycle 25 min. Moderate effort. 30 min. Hard effort.	Rest.	Cycle 15 min. Moderate effort. 35 min. Hard effort.	Rest.	Cycle 25 min. Hard effort.	Rolling hill work: Cycle 25 min. Moderate effort. 25 min. Hard effort.
2 MODERATE	Rest.	Rolling hill work: Cycle 25 min. Moderate effort. 35 min. Hard effort.	Rolling hill work: Cycle 25 min. Moderate effort. 35 min. Hard effort.	Cycle 25 min. Moderate effort.	Rest.	Cycle 30 min. Hard effort.	Rolling hill work: Cycle 25 min. Moderate effort. 30 min. Hard effort.
3 EASY	Rest.	Rolling hill work: Cycle 25 min. Moderate effort. 30 min. Hard effort.	Rest.	Cycle 20 min. Moderate effort.	Rest.	Cycle 25 min. Hard effort.	Rolling hill work: Cycle 25 min. Moderate effort. 25 min. Hard effort.
4 HARD	Rest.	Rolling hill work: Cycle 25 min. Moderate effort. 45 min. Hard effort.	Rolling hill work: Cycle 35 min. Moderate effort. 40 min. Hard effort.	Cycle 35 min. Moderate effort.	Rest.	Cycle 40 min. Hard effort.	Rolling hill work: Cycle 25 min. Moderate effort. 35 min. Hard effort.
5 EASY	Rest.	Rolling hill work: Cycle 25 min. Moderate effort. 40 min. Hard effort.	Game Day.	Cycle 20 min. Moderate effort.	Rest.	Cycle 25 min. Hard effort.	Rolling hill work: Cycle 25 min. Moderate effort. 40 min. Hard effort.
6 HARD	Rest.	Rolling hill work: Cycle 25 min. Moderate effort. 50 min. Hard effort.	Game Day.	Cycle 45 min. Moderate effort.	Rest.	Cycle 50 min. Hard effort.	Rolling hill work: Cycle 25 min. Moderate effort. 50 min. Hard effort.

CYCLING ADVANCED   *10. Laying the Foundation*

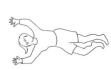

DAY / WEEK	1	Strength Work 2	3	Strength Work 4	5	Strength Work 6	7
1 EASY	Rest.	Cycle 45 min. Hard effort.	Game Day.	Rolling hill work: Cycle 30 min. Moderate effort. 30 min. Hard effort.	Rest.	Rolling hill work: Cycle 30 min. Moderate effort. 40 min. Hard effort.	Cycle 50 min. Hard effort.
2 MODERATE	Rest.	Cycle 55 min. Hard effort.	Game Day.	Rolling hill work: Cycle 30 min. Moderate effort. 40 min. Hard effort.	Rest.	Rolling hill work: Cycle 30 min. Moderate effort. 45 min. Hard effort.	Cycle 60 min. Hard effort.
3 EASY	Rest.	Cycle 50 min. Hard effort.	Game Day.	Rolling hill work: Cycle 30 min. Moderate effort. 35 min. Hard effort.	Rest.	Rolling hill work: Cycle 30 min. Moderate effort. 35 min. Hard effort.	Cycle 55 min. Hard effort.
4 HARD	Rest.	Cycle 55 min. Hard effort.	Game Day.	Rolling hill work: Cycle 30 min. Moderate effort. 45 min. Hard effort.	Rest.	Rolling hill work: Cycle 30 min. Moderate effort. 40 min. Hard effort.	Cycle 60 min. Hard effort.
5 EASY	Rest.	Rolling hill work: Cycle 30 min. Moderate effort. 30 min. Hard effort.	Cycle 50 min. Hard effort.	Game Day.	Rest.	Rolling hill work: Cycle 30 min. Moderate effort. 25 min. Hard effort.	Cycle 55 min. Hard effort.
6 HARD	Rest.	Rolling hill work: Cycle 30 min. Moderate effort. 45 min. Hard effort.	Cycle 60 min. Hard effort.	Game Day.	Rest.	Rolling hill work: Cycle 30 min. Moderate effort. 50 min. Hard effort.	Cycle 65 min. Hard effort.

CYCLING ADVANCED   *11. Building Endurance*

DAY	1	Strength Work 2	3	Strength Work 4	5	Strength Work 6	7
WEEK 1 EASY	Rest.	Cycle 30 min. Moderate effort. 40 min. Hard effort.	Cycle 45 min. Hard effort.	Game Day.	Rest.	Cycle 60 min. Hard effort.	Cycle 30 min. Moderate effort. 40 min. Hard effort.
2 MODERATE	Rest.	Cycle 30 min. Moderate effort. 40 min. Hard effort.	Cycle 65 min. Hard effort.	Game Day.	Rest.	Cycle 70 min. Hard effort.	Cycle 30 min. Moderate effort. 60 min. Hard effort.
3 EASY	Rest.	Cycle 30 min. Moderate effort. 55 min. Hard effort.	Cycle 70 min. Hard effort.	Game Day.	Rest.	Cycle 70 min. Hard effort.	Cycle 30 min. Moderate effort. 55 min. Hard effort.
4 HARD	Rest.	Cycle 85 min. Hard effort.	Cycle 75 min. Hard effort.	Cycle 90 min. Hard effort.	Rest.	Cycle 85 min. Hard effort.	Cycle 90 min. Moderate effort.
5 EASY							
6 HARD							

CYCLING ADVANCED   *12. Achieving Mastery*

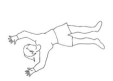

ROWING

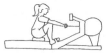

See art, pages 239–267.

TECHNIQUE AND FORM

We wish everyone had access to a boat, but we know that's not realistic. It's also not necessary. For purposes of this workout schedule, we're going to assume that you're rowing indoors on an ergometer, or "erg" for short. The erg simulates the rowing stroke used on the water and puts your muscles through an identical workout. The erg has one advantage over the boat: it's outfitted with a performance monitor—a computer that calculates stroke, elapsed time, split times for 500 meters, and an equivalent distance rowed in meters. No cheating. The data is precisely recorded and ruthlessly fed back to you so you'll know how you're doing. You'll need that feedback because, unlike the real boat, there is no glide, or "run," to give you the sensation of water and its resistance. There's only the expectation of the next stroke's effort. The erg responds to your level of effort. The harder you try, the greater the resistance . . . simulating actual rowing, where the harder you pull the oar against the water, the more effort it takes and the faster the boat goes.

The erg consists of a sliding seat and an oar handle connected by a chain to a flywheel within a drum. The drum has a damper, a lever that opens the drum, which has ten settings similar to the gears on a bicycle. The higher the damper setting, the more air is drawn into the drum as you row, which provides greater resistance against the flywheel, generating greater force—provided the speed of your rowing stroke stays the same. To row effectively on the erg, you must learn to control and regulate your effort. As your technique improves, you'll be able to do more with less effort.

The rowing stroke has four basic parts. The start of the stroke is called the "catch." At the catch, you sit forward in a ready position with your legs bent and your lower legs perpendicular to the floor. Your arms are fully extended; your back is curved; and your shoulders are rolled in front of your hips. As you begin the stroke, push off with your legs while keeping your shoulders forward and your arms straight. You'll feel as if you were pushing the erg away from you with your legs. This portion of the stroke is called the "drive," or "leg drive." Most of the power in the stroke is applied here. After you're more than halfway down the slide, pull with your arms and extend your lower back to draw the oar handle into your solar plexus. This is known as the "finish." Your legs are fully extended and your back, although still curved, is about 15 degrees past vertical. After the finish, you immediately extend your arms forward to the ready position, then contract your abdominals to flex your torso and round your shoulders in front of your hips. Once your hands are past your knees, slowly and with control bend your knees and move the seat down the slide, maintaining the orientation of your shoulders and hips as you prepare to take the next stroke. This is called "recovery."

EQUIPMENT YOU'LL NEED

A watch
A bottle of water
An erg

WHAT TO WEAR

Clothing: Wear anything that's cool, comfortable, and moves with you. You'll also want to wear clothing that wicks sweat away from your body. Because erging is repetitive and you're sitting on a narrow seat, beware of seams, tags, and embellishments that might rub your skin and cause irritation.

Shoes: Running, walking, aerobic, or tennis shoes are fine.

Socks: Socks are optional, but most people appreciate them. They add a layer of protection between your foot and the inside of the shoe, and they put a little extra cushion between the sole of your shoe and the erg. Look for a smooth, snug fit that's free from wrinkles and inside seams. Because even the best socks are an inexpensive investment, go first-class. Purchase athletes' socks that are engineered to "wick" moisture, or absorb sweat away from your foot and provide you with a dryer shoe interior, which will help prevent blistering, skin irritations, and odor. Treat yourself to a clean pair of socks with every workout.

Gloves: Tender hands are a problem with the erg. Wear cycling gloves that are padded in the palms to absorb some of the pressure.

BOREDOM BUSTERS

Listen to music: Portable CD and tape players, and radios with lightweight headsets, are fun. Just make sure that your choice of music is compatible with your planned workout. If you're erging in a facility with other people, be sure you're using a headset that affords you complete privacy. In other words, do

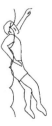

everything possible to keep from imposing (or inflicting) your choice of music—and its accompanying rhythms—on others.

Sign up for an event: Nothing motivates a rower like an upcoming competition or a benefit erg-a-thon. Targeting a specific goal on a specific date puts focus and excitement into even the most wearisome program.

Watch videos: There are videos especially made to simulate movement through an environment, as if you were actually gliding along famous waterways. If you can't find one of these, pop in a movie.

Row for real: While erging is fun, there's something exhilarating about a chance to try out your skills in the real world. Rent or borrow a one-person scull and have a ball. If you can't find a scull, locate a rowboat. It won't provide a refined experience, but you'll get a chance to feel an oar in the water, the wind in your hair, and a smile on your face.

TAKING IT TO THE GYM

Erg

INJURY ALERT

Injuries in rowing and sculling occur most frequently in the knees, which makes sense, as the athlete sits in a very confined position and executes very specific, repetitive movements. The knees, which power this back-and-forth action, track a very specific path. Knee irritation and overuse syndromes are common. Lower back injuries follow knee problems, and are caused by pressure from the seat and exertion from the rowing. In competition, the rowing can be so strenuous that the athlete can even suffer from stress fractures of the ribs from pulling. So much for "Row, row, row your boat *gently* down the stream . . ."

TIPS FROM THE EXPERTS

Rowing and sculling are wonderful exercise, but they aren't perfect by a long shot. Because the tracking of your body is so specific, you're likely to have serious muscle imbalances if you don't supplement your program with a comprehensive strength program. Also, flexibility is critical in holding off the repetitive stress injuries unfortunately inherent in this sport. Having a full range of motion in joints—specifically hips, knees, shoulders, wrists, and back—will help keep you free of irritations and nerve impingements.

Allow yourself plenty of rest during preseason and competition. Warm up adequately before each session.

A final note: please remember to hydrate when you row. (It's especially easy to forget when you're on the water and moving so quickly that sweat evaporates before it has a chance to remind you that you're hot.) Heat problems set in when dehydration lowers the circulating volume of blood and the core temperature starts to rise. Problems manifest themselves in symptoms that include fatigue, lack of coordination, muscle pain and cramping, headache, light-headedness, confusion, disorientation, and fainting. Under extreme circumstances, death can occur. If you feel thirsty, you're already on your way to trouble. Drink early—before thirst sets in—and often. Experts say that water is perfect for short workouts, but a commercial sport fluid-replacement drink is preferable for workouts of more than ninety minutes in duration. With either choice, *cold* is best. We want you to play it cool. Drink.

COMING TO TERMS WITH THE TERMS WE USE IN YOUR SCHEDULE

Easy effort: This is leisurely and conversational. You should be in the minimum range of your target heart rate.

Moderate effort: This is a little harder than easy effort, but still conversational. You should be in the middle range of your target heart rate.

Hard effort: This is exertion in which you'll not be able to easily carry on a conversation. You should be in the higher ranges of your target heart rate.

We developed this program with the assistance of Jim Karanas, the coholder of the world record in the 100-kilometer two-man tandem indoor rowing (5:59:59.0). Today, at age forty-six, Jim has personal bests of 6:32.2 for the 2,000-meter sprint; 8,395 meters for the thirty-minute row; 16,329 meters for the sixty-minute row; and 2:42:51.3 for the marathon. He rows approximately 250 kilometers a week on the erg. Jim is the group exercise and performance training director for Club One, a San Francisco–based chain of fifty-seven commercial and corporate fitness centers located primarily on the West Coast.

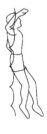

DAY	1	Strength Work 2	3	Strength Work 4	5	Strength Work 6	7
WEEK 1 EASY	Make sure your equipment, shoes, and clothing are in order.	Row 20 min. Easy effort. Damper < 3 Stroke rate < 22	Rest.	Row 20 min. Easy effort. Damper < 3 Stroke rate < 22	Rest.	Row 20 min. Easy effort. Damper < 3 Stroke rate < 22	Row 20 min. Easy effort. Damper < 3 Stroke rate < 22
2 MODERATE	Rest.	Row 30 min. Easy effort. Damper < 3 Stroke rate < 22	Row 35 min. Easy effort. Damper < 3 Stroke rate < 22	Rest.	Row 35 min. Easy effort. Damper < 3 Stroke rate < 22	Rest.	Row 40 min. Easy effort. Damper < 3 Stroke rate < 22
3 EASY							
4 HARD							
5 EASY							
6 HARD							

ROWING BEGINNER *1. Awakening the Body*

ROWING BEGINNER 2. Laying the Foundation

DAY / WEEK	1	Strength Work 2	3	Strength Work 4	5	Strength Work 6	7
1 EASY	Rest.	Row 20 min. Easy effort. Damper < 3. Stroke rate < 22	Row 15 min. Easy effort. Damper < 3. Stroke rate < 22	Row 20 min. Easy effort. Damper < 3. Stroke rate < 22	Rest.	Row 30 min. Easy effort. Damper < 3. Stroke rate < 22	Row 35 min. Easy effort. Damper < 3. Stroke rate < 22
2 MODERATE	Rest.	Row 25 min. Easy effort. Damper < 3. Stroke rate < 22	Row 30 min. Easy effort. Damper < 3. Stroke rate < 22	Rest.	Row 35 min. Easy effort. Damper < 3. Stroke rate < 22	Rest.	Row 40 min. Easy effort. Damper < 3. Stroke rate < 22
3 EASY	Rest.	Row 20 min. Easy effort. Damper < 3. Stroke rate < 22	Rest.	Row 30 min. Easy effort. Damper < 3. Stroke rate < 22	Rest.	Row 30 min. Easy effort. Damper < 3. Stroke rate < 22	Row 20 min. Easy effort. Damper < 3. Stroke rate < 22
4 HARD	Rest.	Row 30 min. Easy effort. Damper < 3. Stroke rate < 22	Row 35 min. Easy effort. Damper < 3. Stroke rate < 22	Row 40 min. Easy effort. Damper < 3. Stroke rate < 22.	Rest.	Row 45 min. Easy effort. Damper < 3. Stroke rate < 22	Row 50 min. Easy effort. Damper < 3. Stroke rate < 22
5 EASY	Rest.	Row 30 min. Easy effort. Damper < 3. Stroke rate < 22	Rest.	Rest.	Row 40 min. Easy effort. Damper < 3. Stroke rate < 22	Rest.	Row 45 min. Easy effort. Damper < 3. Stroke rate < 22
6 HARD	Rest.	Row 30 min. Easy effort. Damper < 3. Stroke rate < 22	Row 35 min. Easy effort. Damper < 3. Stroke rate < 22	Row 30 min. Easy effort. Damper < 3. Stroke rate < 22	Rest.	Row 45 min. Easy effort. Damper < 3. Stroke rate < 22	Row 50 min. Easy effort. Damper < 3. Stroke rate < 22

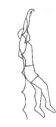

DAY	1	Strength Work 2	3	Strength Work 4	5	Strength Work 6	7
WEEK 1 EASY	Rest.	Row 20 min. Easy effort. Damper < 3 Stroke rate < 22	Row 25 min. Easy effort. Damper < 3 Stroke rate < 22	Rest.	Row 20 min. Easy effort. Damper < 3 Stroke rate < 22	Rest.	Row 25 min. Easy effort. Damper < 3 Stroke rate < 22
2 MODERATE	Rest.	Row 30 min. Easy effort. Damper < 3 Stroke rate < 22	Row 25 min. Easy effort. Damper < 3 Stroke rate < 22	Row 30 min. Easy effort. Damper < 3 Stroke rate < 22	Rest.	Row 30 min. Easy effort. Damper < 3 Stroke rate < 22	Row 35 min. Easy effort. Damper < 3 Stroke rate < 22
3 EASY	Rest.	Row 30 min. Easy effort. Damper < 3 Stroke rate < 22	Row 20 min. Easy effort. Damper < 3 Stroke rate < 22	Rest.	Row 30 min. Easy effort. Damper < 3 Stroke rate < 22	Rest.	Row 30 min. Easy effort. Damper < 3 Stroke rate < 22
4 HARD	Rest.	Row 40 min. Easy effort. Damper < 3 Stroke rate < 22	Row 30 min. Easy effort. Damper < 3 Stroke rate < 22	Row 30 min. Easy effort. Damper < 3 Stroke rate < 22	Rest.	Row 40 min. Easy effort. Damper < 3 Stroke rate < 22	Row 40 min. Easy effort. Damper < 3 Stroke rate < 22
5 EASY	Rest.	Row 40 min. Easy effort. Damper < 3 Stroke rate < 22	Row 30 min. Easy effort. Damper < 3 Stroke rate < 22	Rest.	Row 40 min. Easy effort. Damper < 3 Stroke rate < 22	Rest.	Row 35 min. Easy effort. Damper < 3 Stroke rate < 22
6 HARD	Rest.	Row 50 min. Easy effort. Damper < 3 Stroke rate < 22	Row 40 min. Easy effort. Damper < 3 Stroke rate < 22	Row 50 min. Easy effort. Damper < 3 Stroke rate < 22	Rest.	Row 50 min. Easy effort. Damper < 3 Stroke rate < 22	Row 45 min. Easy effort. Damper < 3 Stroke rate < 22

ROWING BEGINNER   *3. Building Endurance*

ROWING BEGINNER *4. Achieving Mastery*

DAY	1	Strength Work 2	3	Strength Work 4	5	Strength Work 6	7
WEEK 1 EASY	Rest.	Row 30 min. Easy effort. Damper < 3 Stroke rate < 22	Row 30 min. Easy effort. Damper < 4 Stroke rate < 22	Rest.	Row 35 min. Easy effort. Damper < 3 Stroke rate < 22	Row 30 min. Easy effort. Damper < 4 Stroke rate < 22	Row 40 min. Easy effort. Damper < 3 Stroke rate < 22
2 MODERATE	Rest.	Row 40 min. Easy effort. Damper < 4 Stroke rate < 22	Row 30 min. Easy effort. Damper < 4 Stroke rate < 22	Row 50 min. Easy effort. Damper < 3 Stroke rate < 22	Rest.	Row 50 min. Easy effort. Damper < 3 Stroke rate < 22	Row 60 min. Easy effort. Damper < 3 Stroke rate < 22
3 EASY							
4 HARD							
5 EASY							
6 HARD							

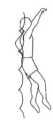

ROWING INTERMEDIATE   5. Awakening the Body

DAY	1	2 Strength Work	3	4 Strength Work	5	6 Strength Work	7
WEEK 1 EASY	Rest.	Row 40 min. Easy effort. Damper < 4 Stroke rate < 22	Row 30 min. Easy effort. Damper < 3 Stroke rate < 22	Row 40 min. Easy effort. Damper < 4 Stroke rate < 22	Rest.	Row 30 min. Easy effort. Damper < 3 Stroke rate < 22	Row 40 min. Easy effort. Damper < 4 Stroke rate < 22
2 MODERATE	Rest.	Row 40 min. Easy effort. Damper < 4 Stroke rate < 22	Row 30 min. Easy effort. Damper < 4 Stroke rate < 22	Row 40 min. Easy effort. Damper < 4 Stroke rate < 22	Rest.	Row 40 min. Easy effort. Damper < 3 Stroke rate < 22	Row 50 min. Easy effort. Damper < 4 Stroke rate < 22
3 EASY							
4 HARD							
5 EASY							
6 HARD							

ROWING INTERMEDIATE 6. Laying the Foundation

DAY / WEEK	1	Strength Work 2	3	Strength Work 4	5	Strength Work 6	7
1 EASY	Rest.	Row 50 min. Moderate effort. Damper < 3 Stroke rate < 22	Rest.	Row 50 min. Easy effort. Damper < 3 Stroke rate < 22	Rest.	Row 50 min. Moderate effort. Damper < 3 Stroke rate < 22	Row 50 min. Easy effort. Damper < 3 Stroke rate < 22
2 MODERATE	Rest.	Row 50 min. Moderate effort. Damper < 3 Stroke rate < 22	Rest.	Row 50 min. Easy effort. Damper < 3 Stroke rate < 22	Rest.	Row 50 min. Moderate effort. Damper < 3 Stroke rate < 22	Row 50 min. Moderate effort. Damper < 3 Stroke rate < 22
3 EASY	Rest.	Row 50 min. Easy effort. Damper < 3 Stroke rate < 22	Rest.	Row 50 min. Easy effort. Damper < 4 Stroke rate 22–24	Rest.	Row 50 min. Easy effort. Damper < 3 Stroke rate < 22	Row 50 min. Moderate effort. Damper < 3 Stroke rate < 22
4 HARD	Rest.	Row 50 min. Moderate effort. Damper < 4 Stroke rate 22–24	Rest.	Row 50 min. Moderate effort. Damper < 4 Stroke rate 22–24	Rest.	Row 50 min. Moderate effort. Damper < 3 Stroke rate < 22	Row 50 min. Moderate effort. Damper < 4 Stroke rate 22–24
5 EASY	Rest.	Row 50 min. Moderate effort. Damper < 4 Stroke rate 22–24	Rest.	Row 50 min. Moderate effort. Damper < 3 Stroke rate < 22	Rest.	Row 50 min. Moderate effort. Damper < 4 Stroke rate 22–24	Row 50 min. Moderate effort. Damper < 3 Stroke rate < 22
6 HARD	Rest.	Row 30 min. Easy effort. Damper < 2 Stroke rate < 22	Rest.	Row 40 min. Moderate effort. Damper < 4 Stroke rate 22–24	Rest.	Row 30 min. Easy effort. Damper < 2 Stroke rate < 22	Row 50 min. Easy effort. Damper < 2 Stroke rate < 22

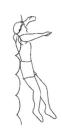

DAY	1	Strength Work 2	3	Strength Work 4	5	Strength Work 6	7
WEEK 1 EASY	Rest.	Row 30 min. Easy effort. Damper < 4 Stroke rate < 24	Rest.	Row 50 min. Easy effort. Damper < 4 Stroke rate < 24	Rest.	Row 30 min. Easy effort. Damper < 4 Stroke rate < 24	Row 40 min. Easy effort. Damper < 4 Stroke rate < 24
2 MODERATE	Rest.	Row 40 min. Moderate effort. Damper < 4 Stroke rate < 24	Row 50 min. Moderate effort. Damper < 4 Stroke rate < 24	Row 40 min. Moderate effort. Damper < 4 Stroke rate < 24	Rest.	Row 40 min. Moderate effort. Damper < 4 Stroke rate < 24	Row 50 min. Moderate effort. Damper < 4 Stroke rate < 24
3 EASY	Rest.	Row 40 min. Easy effort. Damper < 4 Stroke rate < 24	Rest.	Row 50 min. Easy effort. Damper < 4 Stroke rate < 24	Rest.	Row 40 min. Easy effort. Damper < 4 Stroke rate < 24	Row 50 min. Easy effort. Damper < 4 Stroke rate < 24
4 HARD	Rest.	Row 50 min. Moderate effort. Damper < 4 Stroke rate < 24	Row 40 min. Moderate effort. Damper < 4 Stroke rate < 24	Row 50 min. Moderate effort. Damper < 4 Stroke rate 22–24	Rest.	Row 40 min. Moderate effort. Damper < 4 Stroke rate 22–24	Row 50 min. Moderate effort. Damper < 4 Stroke rate 22–24
5 EASY	Rest.	Row 40 min. Moderate effort. Damper < 4 Stroke rate < 24	Rest.	Row 30 min. Moderate effort. Damper < 4 Stroke rate < 24	Rest.	Row 30 min. Moderate effort. Damper < 4 Stroke rate < 24	Row 40 min. Moderate effort. Damper < 4 Stroke rate < 24
6 HARD	Rest.	Row 50 min. Moderate effort. Damper < 4 Stroke rate < 24	Rest.	Row 50 min. Moderate effort. Damper < 4 Stroke rate < 24	Rest.	Row 50 min. Moderate effort. Damper < 4 Stroke rate < 24	Row 50 min. Moderate effort. Damper < 4 Stroke rate < 24

ROWING INTERMEDIATE   *7. Building Endurance*

DAY	1	Strength Work 2	3	Strength Work 4	5	Strength Work 6	7
WEEK 1 EASY	Rest.	Row 30 min. Moderate effort. Damper < 4 Stroke rate < 24	Rest.	Row 40 min. Moderate effort. Damper < 2 Stroke rate 22–24	Rest.	Row 30 min. Moderate effort. Damper < 4 Stroke rate < 24	Row 40 min. Moderate effort. Damper < 2 Stroke rate 22–24
2 MODERATE	Rest.	Row 40 min. Moderate effort. Damper < 4 Stroke rate < 24	Row 30 min. Moderate effort. Damper < 4 Stroke rate < 24	Row 40 min. Moderate effort. Damper < 4 Stroke rate < 24	Rest.	Row 40 min. Moderate effort. Damper < 4 Stroke rate < 24	Row 50 min. Moderate effort. Damper < 2 Stroke rate < 24
3 EASY	Rest.	Row 40 min. Moderate effort. Damper < 4 Stroke rate < 24	Rest.	Row 40 min. Moderate effort. Damper < 2 Stroke rate 22–24	Rest.	Row 30 min. Moderate effort. Damper < 4 Stroke rate < 24	Row 40 min. Moderate effort. Damper < 2 Stroke rate 22–24
4 HARD	Rest.	Row 30 min. Hard effort. Damper < 4 Stroke rate 22–24	Row 40 min. Moderate effort. Damper < 4 Stroke rate 22–24	Row 30 min. Hard effort. Damper < 4 Stroke rate 22–24	Rest.	Row 30 min. Moderate effort. Damper < 4 Stroke rate 22–24	Row 40 min. Hard effort. Damper < 4 Stroke rate 22–24
5 EASY							
6 HARD							

ROWING INTERMEDIATE   *8. Achieving Mastery*

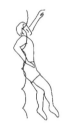

DAY	1	Strength Work 2	3	Strength Work 4	5	Strength Work 6	7
WEEK 1 EASY	Rest.	Row 30 min. Moderate effort. Damper < 2 Stroke rate < 24	Rest.	Row 40 min. Moderate effort. Damper < 2 Stroke rate < 24	Rest.	Row 30 min. Easy effort. Damper < 2 Stroke rate < 24	Row 40 min. Moderate effort. Damper < 2 Stroke rate < 24
2 MODERATE	Rest.	Row 30 min. Hard effort. Damper < 4 Stroke rate 22–24	Rest.	Row 40 min. Hard effort. Damper < 4 Stroke rate 22–24	Rest.	Row 30 min. Moderate effort. Damper < 4 Stroke rate 22–24	Row 40 min. Hard effort. Damper < 4 Stroke rate 22–24
3 EASY							
4 HARD							
5 EASY							
6 HARD							

ROWING ADVANCED   9. Awakening the Body

DAY WEEK	1	Strength Work 2	3	Strength Work 4	5	Strength Work 6	7
1 EASY	Rest.	Row 40 min. Moderate effort. Damper < 4. Stroke rate 22–24	Rest.	Row 30 min. Moderate effort. Damper < 4. Stroke rate 22–24	Rest.	Row 30 min. Moderate effort. Damper < 4. Stroke rate 22–24	Row 40 min. Hard effort. Damper < 4. Stroke rate 22–24
2 MODERATE	Rest.	Row 40 min. Hard effort. Damper < 4. Stroke rate < 25	Row 30 min. Hard effort. Damper < 4. Stroke rate < 25	Row 40 min. Hard effort. Damper < 4. Stroke rate < 25	Rest.	Row 30 min. Hard effort. Damper < 4. Stroke rate < 25	Row 40 min. Hard effort. Damper < 4. Stroke rate < 25
3 EASY	Rest.	Row 40 min. Moderate effort. Damper < 4. Stroke rate 22–24	Rest.	Row 30 min. Moderate effort. Damper < 4. Stroke rate 22–24	Rest.	Row 30 min. Moderate effort. Damper < 4. Stroke rate 22–24	Row 40 min. Hard effort. Damper < 4. Stroke rate 22–24
4 HARD	Rest.	Row 40 min. Hard effort. Damper < 2. Stroke rate < 25	Row 40 min. Hard effort. Damper < 2. Stroke rate < 25	Row 40 min. Hard effort. Damper < 4. Stroke rate < 25	Rest.	Row 40 min. Hard effort. Damper < 2. Stroke rate < 25	Row 45 min. Hard effort. Damper < 2. Stroke rate < 25
5 EASY	Rest.	Row 40 min. Hard effort. Damper < 4. Stroke rate 22–24	Game Day.	Row 30 min. Moderate effort. Damper < 4. Stroke rate 22–24	Rest.	Row 40 min. Hard effort. Damper < 4. Stroke rate 22–24	Row 45 min. Moderate effort. Damper < 4. Stroke rate 22–24
6 HARD	Rest.	Row 45 min. Hard effort. Damper < 2. Stroke rate < 25	Game Day.	Row 40 min. Hard effort. Damper < 2. Stroke rate < 25	Rest.	Row 45 min. Hard effort. Damper < 2. Stroke rate < 25	Row 55 min. Hard effort. Damper < 2. Stroke rate < 25

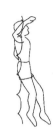

ROWING ADVANCED   10. Laying the Foundation

DAY	1	2 (Strength Work)	3	4 (Strength Work)	5	6 (Strength Work)	7 (Strength Work)
WEEK 1 EASY	Rest.	Row 45 min. Moderate effort. Damper < 2. Stroke rate < 22	Game Day.	Row 55 min. Hard effort. Damper < 2. Stroke rate < 22	Rest.	Row 45 min. Moderate effort. Damper < 2. Stroke rate < 22	Row 50 min. Hard effort. Damper < 2. Stroke rate < 22
2 MODERATE	Rest.	Row 55 min. Hard effort. Damper < 2. Stroke rate < 24	Game Day.	Row 55 min. Hard effort. Damper < 2. Stroke rate < 24	Rest.	Row 45 min. Hard effort. Damper < 2. Stroke rate < 24	Row 55 min. Hard effort. Damper < 2. Stroke rate < 24
3 EASY	Rest.	Row 55 min. Moderate effort. Damper < 2. Stroke rate < 22	Game Day.	Row 45 min. Moderate effort. Damper < 2. Stroke rate < 22	Rest.	Row 50 min. Moderate effort. Damper < 2. Stroke rate < 22	Row 55 min. Moderate effort. Damper < 2. Stroke rate < 22
4 HARD	Rest.	Row 55 min. Hard effort. Damper < 2. Stroke rate < 25	Game Day.	Row 60 min. Hard effort. Damper < 2. Stroke rate < 25	Rest.	Row 55 min. Hard effort. Damper < 2. Stroke rate < 25	Row 65 min. Hard effort. Damper < 2. Stroke rate < 25
5 EASY	Rest.	Row 55 min. Moderate effort. Damper < 2. Stroke rate < 22	Row 40 min. Moderate effort. Damper < 2. Stroke rate < 22	Game Day.	Rest.	Row 55 min. Moderate effort. Damper < 2. Stroke rate < 22	Row 60 min. Moderate effort. Damper < 2. Stroke rate < 22
6 HARD	Rest.	Row 65 min. Hard effort. Damper < 4. Stroke rate < 25	Row 60 min. Hard effort. Damper < 4. Stroke rate < 25	Game Day.	Rest.	Row 65 min. Hard effort. Damper < 4. Stroke rate < 25	Row 70 min. Hard effort. Damper < 4. Stroke rate < 25

ROWING ADVANCED   *11. Building Endurance*

DAY	1	Strength Work 2	3	Strength Work 4	5	Strength Work 6	7
WEEK 1 EASY	Rest.	Row 55 min. Hard effort. Damper < 4. Stroke rate < 25	Row 30 min. Easy effort. Damper < 2. Stroke rate < 22	Game Day.	Rest.	Row 55 min. Hard effort. Damper < 4. Stroke rate < 25	Row 60 min. Hard effort. Damper < 4. Stroke rate < 25
2 MODERATE	Rest.	Row 55 min. Hard effort. Damper < 4. Stroke rate < 25	Row 60 min. Hard effort. Damper < 4. Stroke rate < 25	Game Day.	Rest.	Row 65 min. Hard effort. Damper < 4. Stroke rate < 25	Row 70 min. Hard effort. Damper < 4. Stroke rate < 25
3 EASY	Rest.	Row 60 min. Hard effort. Damper < 4. Stroke rate < 25	Row 30 min. Easy effort. Damper < 2. Stroke rate < 22	Game Day.	Rest.	Row 60 min. Hard effort. Damper < 4. Stroke rate < 25	Row 55 min. Hard effort. Damper < 4. Stroke rate < 25
4 HARD	Rest.	Row 70 min. Hard effort. Damper < 4. Stroke rate < 25	Row 60 min. Hard effort. Damper < 4. Stroke rate < 25	Row 70 min. Hard effort. Damper < 4. Stroke rate < 25	Rest.	Row 60 min. Hard effort. Damper < 4. Stroke rate < 25	Row 75 min. Hard effort. Damper < 4. Stroke rate < 25
5 EASY							
6 HARD							

ROWING ADVANCED   12. *Achieving Mastery*

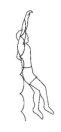

PART FOUR

The Enduring Life

11.

Keeping Your Health from Going Up in Smoke

Generally, when we design a health and fitness program for an aspiring athlete, we come up with a list of things to do and a schedule. In working with a smoker, we start with a shorter list and a tighter schedule: stop smoking. Do it right this second.

If there is one thing about which we are unapologetically militant, it is the clear conviction that smoking is a killer and has no place in an intelligent, healthy person's life. As former U.S. Surgeon General C. Everett Koop, M.D., said to the smokers of America, "If you have a spouse who's nagging you at home to quit, children who suggest that you're going to die if you don't, and then your boss says you can't smoke at the worksite, that's a pretty good indication that it's time to try to quit." But quitting is easier said than done. Ask the 15.7 million Americans who tried to quit last year and failed, and the relatively few—1.3 million—who succeeded.

There is no question that smoking cigarettes is a tough habit to kick. Indeed, nicotine, the addictive ingredient in tobacco, has been compared to heroin for its ferocious hold on victims. But another attempt is worth the effort if it will break you free from smoking.

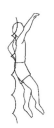

Smoking is the most preventable cause of death in our society, responsible for one out of five deaths in the United States. Half of those deaths cut lives short by twenty to twenty-five years. Smoking is responsible for 87 percent of all lung cancers. Lung cancer is only one of the long list of diseases—both debilitating and fatal—that are caused by smoking. People who smoke more than twenty-five cigarettes per day (a little over a pack) are six hundred times more likely to suffer heart attacks than nonsmokers. Smoking is directly associated with 29 percent of all cancer deaths: cancers of the mouth, pharynx, esophagus, pancreas, cervix, kidney, and bladder. Smoking is a major risk factor in cardiovascular disease and is associated with colds, gastric ulcers, chronic bronchitis, and emphysema. As you enter your middle years, the risks increase exponentially.

JUST HOW FAR HAVE WOMEN COME?

Cigarette manufacturers sing the praises of women smokers: "You've come a long way, baby!" And it's absolutely true, as long as you don't look too closely at which way women are going. Today, in spite of the well-known and indisputable health risks associated with smoking, more women than ever are lighting up. The American Lung Association reports that 22.2 million American women are smokers. Sadly, the disparity between male and female deaths from lung cancer is narrowing, and the number of women with the disease is increasing. Smoking is proving to be an equal-opportunity killer. Some experts predict that cigarette smoking alone will eventually wipe out the seven-year longevity edge that women now enjoy over men. The U.S. Surgeon General has declared that cigarette smoking is the number-one hazard in women's health today.

If you are a woman, cigarette smoking has insidious side effects specific to your gender. The more cigarettes you smoke and the longer you smoke, the more likely you are to develop cervical cancer. You are more likely to develop peptic ulcers. Hopeful mothers-to-be who smoke have about a 46 percent higher infertility rate than nonsmokers because cigarette smoking lowers a woman's estrogen levels. Once pregnant, smokers are at increased risk of suffering a miscarriage or stillbirth. You also risk potentially serious complications of pregnancy, including bleeding and premature rupture of the amniotic sac. You may deliver babies with deficits in growth, intellectual and emotional development, and behavior. You could experience menopause one to two years earlier than a nonsmoker. You have increased risk of osteoporosis because of lower estrogen levels and lighter body weight. You are more likely to suffer from incontinence (loss of bladder control). You are at increased risk of developing breast cancer. And smoking makes your skin age, causing premature and severe wrinkling.

CIGARETTE SMOKING ISN'T JUST ABOUT YOU

Cigarette smoking doesn't ruin just *your* health. It is damaging to those healthy nonsmokers who live and breathe around you. Passive smoking (or breathing secondhand smoke) puts your loved ones at risk of developing lung cancer and heart disease. Additionally, it can aggravate existing asthma, chronic bronchitis, and allergies in nonsmokers. If you have children, you are putting them at risk of respiratory infections and problems.

But the most dangerous thing about smoking is that it makes you blind to all of the above.

YES, YES, YOU'VE HEARD IT ALL BEFORE, AND YET . . .

It's true that quitting smoking is very difficult. But it's not nearly so difficult as dying or harming someone you love. So now is the time to quit. Recent studies in smoking cessation programs and advances in nicotine substitutes are making it easier than ever for you to take control and quit.

How you quit seems to be a matter of personal choice. There is no one answer for everyone. Depending on your tastes and needs, you may choose to quit on your own, or join a group to help you through the tough times; you may quit abruptly, or taper off; or you may choose to use a nicotine substitute, or just let nature take its course.

THE SUCCESSFUL METHODS

On Your Own or in a Group?

On your own: The U.S. Department of Health and Human Services recently reported that 90 percent of successful quitters used a self-help strategy. Organizations such as the American Lung Association and the American Cancer Society have educational materials and self-guided programs to help you.

Clinics: If you need the support of a professional or a group of peers, you should try a smoking-cessation clinic. Be prepared for a commitment of time and possible expense. Long-term outcomes are reported to be favorable.

Cold Turkey or Gradually Quitting

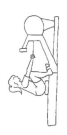

Cold turkey: Most programs (self-help and clinic-based) advocate going cold turkey. This means that you wake up one morning, smoke your last cigarette, crumple up the empty pack, throw it in the trash, and walk away from smoking forever. Just like that. Of course, you will have to suffer abrupt withdrawal, but unpleasant symptoms are short-term and can be eased with nicotine substitutes—some even available over the counter.

Gradual cessation: Studies indicate that quitting gradually—cutting down a little more every day until you have quit smoking completely—is statistically more successful than quitting all at once. The trick is to smoke on a schedule, having a cigarette by appointment whether or not you want one. This forces you to break your smoking patterns and weakens your habits. You increase the time between cigarettes until your next cigarette just never happens.

TO SUBSTITUTE NICOTINE OR NOT?

Nicotine substitutes: The symptoms of withdrawal can be eased considerably by the use of substitutes that deliver doses of gradually reduced nicotine while you concentrate on modifying your behavior and get used to life without cigarettes. Research suggests that these substitutes are most effective when used in conjunction with another program that includes counseling and follow-up. Although your physician can prescribe a good nicotine substitute, you can also purchase some products without prescription. If you choose an over-the-counter version of a nicotine substitute, using it under a medical professional's supervision is a good idea, because they can have side effects.

Nicotine gum: This chewing gum delivers nicotine to your system as you chew or hold the gum in your mouth. The dosages are adjusted for the numbers of cigarettes you used to smoke per day. The idea is to chew a piece of gum every one to two hours for the first few weeks, and then adjust to one piece every two to four hours, and then finish your program with one piece every four to eight hours. The programs generally run eight to ten weeks.

Nicotine patch: This is a small adhesive "transdermal" patch impregnated with nicotine. It delivers a steady dose of nicotine that passes from the patch through your skin and into your body. You may wear one all the time or take it off at bedtime. In a program that lasts approximately ten weeks, you wear patches with diminishing dosages of nicotine until each dose is so small that you can discontinue use without effect.

Nicotine spray: Reportedly more powerful than gums or patches, this is nicotine in a pump bottle from which a smoker inhales to ward off cravings. Sprays are available by prescription only, and are limited to use no longer than six months.

New on the horizon is a combination of protocols called the "one-two chemical punch." Scientists are using a nicotine patch in combination with mecamylamine, a blood pressure medication that blocks the effects of nicotine and makes cigarettes taste bad. Nicotine produces its pleasurable effects by binding to receptors, specific sites in brain cells. When the two drugs are used together, the nicotine and mecamylamine both bind to receptors, but the mecamylamine blocks nicotine's pleasure trigger. The net effect is that nicotine dampens the craving and mecamylamine takes all the fun out of smoking. Other products presently in development and soon to be available are nicotine inhalers and nicotine tablets, to be held under the tongue.

WILL I GAIN WEIGHT?

Maybe. But so what? Studies have found that about 70 percent of the people who quit smoking gain an average of five pounds in the first month after quitting. Ten percent lose weight and 20 percent stay the same. One reason for a little gain is that nicotine is a powerful stimulant that accelerates the body's metabolism—the rate at which you burn calories. When you quit smoking, your body slows down. If you don't cut calories or increase your physical activity to offset the difference, you will gain a little weight. Another reason is that craving a cigarette is often confused with a hunger pang. You're used to putting something into your mouth, so you substitute with food.

Giving up smoking *and* having to diet at the same time are a lot to deal with at one time, particularly if you are one of many people who took up smoking to control their weight. The truth is that the health benefits are worth the effort. Weight gain can be prevented or reversed with some simple strategies. Substitute low calorie foods for cigarettes. Try sugarless gum or hard candy, raw vegetables, or air-popped popcorn. Avoid eating too much sugar in your diet. Drink plenty of water to more quickly leach the nicotine from your body's tissues and to keep you adequately hydrated. And get moving. Exercise is a wonderful way to burn calories, occupy your mind, throw the brakes on depression, and start your journey back to good health.

WHAT ABOUT FILTERS, SMOKELESS TOBACCO, CIGARS, OR PIPES?

Forget them. Tobacco, no matter how you use it, is deadly.

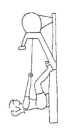

THE TIME TO QUIT IS RIGHT NOW

It has never been easier to quit. Smoking cessation programs—both self-help and clinic-based—have been around so long that they are highly developed and

CIGARETTES: A LETHAL CHEMICAL COMBINATION IN EVERY PUFF

Nicotine is addictive, but it's not the only culprit in a cigarette. There are four thousand chemicals in each puff. Forty-three of them are known to cause cancer, and many others are toxic or damaging to the genes. Here are a few on the deadly list:

- Acetone: paint stripper
- Ammonia: powerful cleaning product
- Arsenic: poison
- Benzene: toxin found in gasoline and so damaging that, when found in trace amounts in some bottles, it forced the recall of Perrier mineral water
- Butane: lighter fluid
- Cadmium: element used in rechargeable batteries
- Carbon monoxide: the poisonous emission from car exhaust
- Cyanide: rat poison
- DDT: insecticide banned in the United States
- Formaldehyde: chemical used to embalm corpses
- Lead: toxic metal
- Methanol: jet fuel
- Methyl isocyanate: poison gas that killed two thousand people in India when it was accidentally released from a Union Carbide factory
- Naphthalene: active ingredient in mothballs
- Nicotine: addictive ingredient in tobacco, also an insecticide
- Polonium 210: cancerous radioactive element

Source: The American Lung Association of Arizona/New Mexico

have proven records for success. Nicotine substitutes are available over the counter. Weight-control programs and fitness centers are easily accessible and inexpensive; educational materials are plentiful and simple to understand. Society is trying to encourage you by giving you the clear message that your smoking is not acceptable where healthy people gather, work, and play. Insurance companies are offering you economic incentives to quit.

Most important, you are now an athlete. And athletes do not smoke.

SOME TIPS FOR QUITTING

1. Keep oral substitutes handy: carrots, pickles, apples, celery, raisins, and gum.

2. Take ten deep breaths and hold the last one while lighting a match. Exhale slowly and blow out the match. Pretend it is a cigarette and put it out in an ashtray.

3. Take a shower, or a bath if possible.

4. Learn to relax quickly and deeply. Make yourself limp, visualize a soothing, pleasing situation, and get away from it all for a moment. Concentrate on that peaceful image and nothing else.

5. Light incense or a candle instead of a cigarette.

6. Never allow yourself to think that just one won't hurt, because it will.

Source: The American Cancer Society

WHAT HAPPENS WHEN YOU STOP SMOKING

WITHIN TWENTY MINUTES

- Blood pressure drops to normal
- Pulse rate drops to normal
- Body temperature of hands and feet increases to normal

WITHIN EIGHT HOURS

- Carbon monoxide level in blood drops to normal
- Oxygen level in blood increases to normal

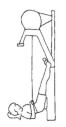

WITHIN TWENTY-FOUR HOURS

- Risk of heart attack decreases

WITHIN FORTY-EIGHT HOURS

- Nerve endings start to regrow in your nose
- Ability to smell and taste is enhanced

WITHIN SEVENTY-TWO HOURS

- Bronchial tubes relax, making breathing easier
- Lung capacity increases—physical activity is easier

BETWEEN TWO WEEKS AND THREE MONTHS

- Circulation improves
- Walking becomes easier
- Lung function increases up to 30 percent

BETWEEN ONE AND NINE MONTHS

- Coughing, sinus congestion, fatigue, shortness of breath decrease
- Body's overall energy level increases
- Cilia regrow in lungs, increasing ability to handle mucus, clean lungs, reduce infection

AT FIVE YEARS

- Lung cancer death rate drops

AT TEN YEARS

- Lung cancer death rate for average smoker drops to twelve deaths per hundred thousand—almost the rate of nonsmokers
- Precancerous cells are replaced
- Other cancers—such as those of the mouth, larynx, esophagus, bladder, kidney, and pancreas—decrease (remember, there are forty-three chemicals in tobacco smoke that cause cancer)

Source: The American Lung Association of Arizona/New Mexico

INTERNET SOURCES FOR SMOKING-CESSATION PROGRAMS

American Cancer Society
http://www.cancer.org/cancerinfo/res—home.asp?ct=26

National Cancer Institute
http://www.nci.nih.gov/

American Heart Association
National Center
http://www.americanheart.org/

Office on Smoking and Health
Centers for Disease Control and Prevention
http://www.cdc.gov/tobacco/

American Lung Association
http://www.lungusa.org/

12.
Fueling Your Training

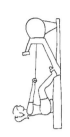

If there is one theme that dominates the design of training programs for our beginning athletes, it's *food*. What do I eat? When do I eat it? How much is enough and how much is too much? Bookshelves and magazine racks lob an endless barrage of promises and possibilities: change your diet and change your life. We like to remember one friend who bought a magazine, on the cover of which was a firm guarantee that she could LOSE 10 POUNDS BY CHRISTMAS! The problem was that although the magazine had been on the shelf since before Thanksgiving, she had not purchased it until December tenth. We could barely contain our merriment as we pointed out that she should have waited even longer to buy the magazine. After all, the editors had promised ten pounds off by Christmas (forget the timetable!), and there was no need to start too early. Why cut short festive holiday eating and partying? In fact, we suggested, wait until December 23! All joking aside, you *can* change your diet and change your life . . . but not in a few short days. We hate to disappoint anyone (especially our friend who wanted ten pounds off by Christmas), but there's no magic involved. As with all aspects of training, diet requires education, discipline, time, and effort.

Generally, when we think of "diet," our minds instantly leap to "weight loss." But in the context of athletic training, we need to make a not-so-subtle shift in thinking. First, a diet is an eating plan. No more. No less. And second, the purpose of a diet is not weight loss (although that might be one possible outcome of an eating plan). A diet is an eating plan designed to provide your body with fuel. Read this paragraph again. And again. Until it is ingrained.

FOOD IS FUEL

Food is one of the raw materials that your body uses to fire muscles, connect nerves, grow, heal, and manufacture things it needs. It's fuel. The better the fuel, the better the outcome of your body's performance. We frequently use the analogy of engineering a finely tuned race car. If we invest a lot of talent and work into making that car run efficiently enough to win every race, the last thing we would do is to fill its tank with low-grade gasoline. Not having the best fuel would undermine all our work and eventually erode the engine parts. The same is true of the body you're working hard to condition. Your body deserves the best fuel in order to do the job you're training it to do. It makes no sense to fill your own tank with low-grade food . . . or worse.

When we and our athletes choose food, we do so based on its nutritional value. Day by day, meal by meal, snack by snack, we evaluate the benefit of each bite and balance it against our needs. If it doesn't serve our purposes, it doesn't make its way into our kitchens. We'll admit that we enjoy eating, but as athletes, our relationship to food is inarguably different from that of "recreational eaters." Food is our fuel. Being delicious and looking good are secondary (and sometimes unnecessary) benefits. If we can do one simple thing—change your attitude toward food so that you, too, think of it as fuel—then you'll be well on your way to eating like an athlete.

WHEN FOOD IS FOOD, AND WHEN IT'S NOT

A few years ago we were invited by our friend (and coauthor) Bev Browning to work on a complicated fitness project. To ensure focus on the work and to guard against interruptions, we left the safety and security of our Manhattan clinic and went to a retreat (without phones!) deep in the wilds of central Florida. Because our dietary requirements and preferences varied widely, each of us brought our own food for the week and cooked separately, but gathered at mealtime to relax and talk. As frequently happens, conversation one night turned to the Wharton diet . . . and the oft-asked questions about life without chocolate: What's it like? Is it as empty and meaningless as it appears? And why do we bother to live at all? During one of our shared meals and the discussions regarding diet, Bev admitted that she struggled with getting weight off and keeping her energy up. She asked our opinion. We made a quick observation after having eaten most meals with her for a few days and seeing what she brought to the table. In spite of her low-calorie meals, most of the calories she ingested were for fun, not nutrition: sugar-free flavored gelatins, fat-free crackers, fat-free cookies, diet soda, and lettuce with fat-free dressings. Bev was eating for entertainment: choosing edible things (notice we did not say "food") that tasted good. But she had completely lost sight of the concept that food is fuel. Her body was starving for nutrition. Constant hunger was her body's demand for fuel. Low energy was the result of Bev's inability to properly interpret a case of self-imposed starvation. The combination of constant hunger and low energy had flattened her metabolism to the point where her body was incredibly efficient at conserving the few useful calories she ate. It was hanging on to each and every morsel. No wonder she was dragging and couldn't lose weight. Before you think we're picking on Bev, let us tell you that she's typical of well-intentioned and intelligent, yet uniformed, people. By the way, you should have seen Bev's face when we suggested that her problem with the inability to lose weight would be easily remedied if she ate more food. She laughed right out loud. We stopped her in mid-guffaw. We pointedly repeated the words "More *food.*" Real food. Calorie-packed food. Nutrition-rich food. Food as fuel. Bev stopped laughing and went shopping.

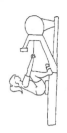

Food (and only food) is the key to a healthy diet. Once you've mastered the concept of food as fuel, then your job will be to design a balanced diet, and to balance your nutritional requirements against your calorie and fat intake. As mounting evidence by researchers links diet to disease prevention and treatment, you can be certain that what you eat has a direct effect on your health, as well as your athletic performance. A good, balanced diet reduces the risk of premature death from our biggest killers—heart disease; hypertension; some cancers such as endometrial, breast, and colon; stroke; and non-insulin-dependent diabetes.

Although we are not going to focus on weight loss, being able to maintain a stable and healthy weight is another compelling reason to get a handle on your diet. There is alarming evidence that the pounds you put on in your middle years are more hazardous to your health than extra weight you've carried since childhood.

DESIGNING AN EATING PLAN JUST FOR YOU

So how do we design a good diet for you? There are thousands of books on the subject and an entire profession—the American Dietetic Association—devoted to laying out specific guidelines. We can't give you hard and fast rules for *The Perfect Diet.* Each of us is unique, with specific needs and tastes. But if you want a few simple suggestions that will make big differences immediately, here they are:

1. Make certain that 99 percent of what you eat is *food.*

2. Cut down sugar.

3. Increase fiber.

4. Cut down fat.

5. Drink water.

HOW TO BEGIN

You can't decide to eat more or less of something unless you know how much of that something you're eating now. It's important to have a starting point. To begin to design your diet, you need to take a hard look at your eating habits. You need to know two things:

1. What are you eating right now?

2. Do you see food as fuel, or does it serve other purposes in your life?

One good way to evaluate your diet is to keep an eating diary for a week or so. Write down every bite you eat and every drop you drink, and make note of the times of day and how you felt about the experience. For example: *"3:00— Grabbed a candy bar and diet soda. Starving even though had lunch. Nervous about presentation at 4. Felt better after eating."* At the end of your week of record-keeping, examine your diet closely, harshly, and honestly. Make note of empty calories (like Bev's edibles for fun), identify fat, sugar, and fiber, and look for balance. Equally important, take a look at your emotional connection to food. Notice how often you drink, how much you drink, and what you choose. You just might be shocked by what you discover.

Another way we evaluate an athlete's diet is to conduct a surprise inspection of his or her kitchen. In addition to examining the contents of every cupboard and the refrigerator, we look for clues regarding an athlete's satisfaction with his or her diet and confidence in the choices made. Interestingly, we've discovered that the more unsure athletes are about their diets, the more likely they are to load up on supplements. The numbers of potions and pills are in direct proportion to uncertainty. If we see a few supplements, we can assume the athlete is confident his or her diet is a good one. Up to ten supplements, the athlete might be on shaky ground. More than ten supplements (including those that have names that sound vaguely intergalactic and exotically mystical), the athlete has no confidence in the diet at all and is relying on supplements to do the job that food should be doing. By the way, we support the use of vitamins, minerals, and herbal supplements as long as they are used in conjunction with a good diet.

When we inspect an athlete's kitchen, we show up with large plastic bags. Our intention is to teach the athlete about food (specifically the difference between an "edible" and real food), and then do him or her a favor by removing useless edibles and leaving the food. We have been known to strip a fully stocked kitchen down to two items. (By the way, we donate the edibles to shelters when we determine the donation is appropriate. We think there's some stuff that *no one* should eat, so it goes into the garbage or the composting bin.)

You don't need a plastic-bag-toting Wharton to evaluate your kitchen. You can do it yourself. Take this checklist into your kitchen and have at it.

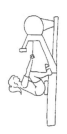

THE SEVEN-POINT REFRIGERATOR RATER

Let's measure your respect for food:

1. TRUE/FALSE: I have things in my refrigerator I can't identify (and really wouldn't want to).

2. TRUE/FALSE: I have things in my refrigerator I can probably identify because they vaguely resemble the original items in spite of differences in shape or color. (Foil swans don't count.)

3. TRUE/FALSE: I have things in my refrigerator that are out of date.

4. TRUE/FALSE: I store food in the refrigerator on designated shelves or in drawers.

5. TRUE/FALSE: I know everything in the refrigerator and intend to serve it within a short period of time.

6. Which of these items do you have the most of?

    A. Things that will go sour if they are not kept cold.

    B. Things that will spoil if they are not kept cold.

    C. Things that will last longer if they are kept cold.

    D. Things I'm trying to hide.

    E. Things I have no place else to store.

    F. What is this stuff???

7. Item by item, answer this question: If Jim and Phil were looking over my shoulder right now, would I frantically try to cover up this stuff, deny it was mine, and wonder out loud (and indignantly) how it got here?

How your refrigerator rates:

1. If you answered TRUE, you are probably not respectful of your food and probably waste a great deal of money by purchasing things you never get around to eating. You might be a food "collector," a person who needs the security of owning food whether or not you ever serve it.

2. If you answered TRUE, you are probably fairly respectful of food, but you think of food as a personal possession (not fuel with a short shelf life). You probably can't stand to waste anything or throw anything away. But before you pat yourself on the back for being frugal, realize that there is something decidedly odd about hanging on to food while you watch it slowly deteriorate. Ask yourself why you do it.

3. If you answered TRUE, you are probably respectful of food, but time gets away from you. You do not plan or budget well. Also, you might be an eternal optimist, one who believes that if it looks good and smells good, it must be good . . . no matter that the product has last year's date on it. Besides, aging improves flavor, right? A good bet is that your refrigerator is loaded with processed food, because you have not learned to work with fresh, live food.

4. If you answered TRUE, you are respectful of food. You recognize that the refrigerator has chilling zones that are specific to storage of different foods, and take advantage of that feature. You're caring for your food and organizing it.

5. If you answered TRUE, you are very respectful of food. You plan and budget well, and tend to make rational decisions regarding your diet. You minimize waste and maximize the benefits of your diet. Your relationship to food is disciplined.

6. Which of these items do you have the most of?

If you answered:

    A. Things that will go sour if they are not kept cold: You probably have a lot of fat in your diet. You're noticing dairy. High fat. Low fiber.

    B. Things that will spoil if they are not kept cold: You have a lot of protein and mixed foods (like casseroles that include different food groups) in your diet. High fat. Low fiber.

    C. Things that will last longer if they are kept cold: You have a lot of live foods in your diet (like fruits and vegetables). High fiber. Good for you. Or you might be noticing sweet things (like pastry). High sugar. Uh-oh.

    D. Things I'm trying to hide: Your relationship with food is a complicated one, balanced somewhere between compulsion and guilt. You have a lot of work to do before you'll be able to see food as fuel, and not some forbidden pleasure.

    E. Things I have no place else to store: There's nothing wrong with cold storage and keeping a kitchen tidy by putting food out of

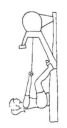

sight, but you want to be certain that you're not crowding out valuable shelf space to store your canned tuna collection.

F. **What is this stuff???:** You need to take a large plastic bag and get rid of everything you can't identify. If you'll never eat that stuff, what's the point of storing it? Besides, who knows what's going on in your refrigerator after that little light goes off?

7. Item by item, you need to take a look at the contents of your refrigerator. Now that you're in "athlete" mode, you're looking for *food.* Pretend that we are with you. Can you defend the edible with a Wharton breathing down your neck and squinting at your little tinfoiled treasure? Is it food? Will your body be able to use it for fuel? Would you serve it to one of us? If you can answer yes to those questions, then keep the food, with our congratulations. If the edible on your refrigerator shelf is not food, then it needs to be compost. Right now.

THE SEVEN-POINT CUPBOARD DISCOVERY

1. TRUE/FALSE: I have more food in my cupboard than I do in my refrigerator.

2. TRUE/FALSE: I have food in my cupboard more than four months old.

3. TRUE/FALSE: I have food in my cupboard more than four years old, and frankly I'm not even sure where it is, but I know it's there. Somewhere.

4. TRUE/FALSE: I use a can opener more than I use a vegetable peeler.

5. TRUE/FALSE: I know how to season with herbs and spices. In fact, I consider myself to be pretty talented at dressing up a dish.

6. Rank the following clusters of foods you have stored in your cupboard. A rank of one (1) means that you have more of this than anything else. A rank of ten (10) means that you have little or none of this.

_____ A. Edibles in cellophane or plastic bags, such as packaged chips

_____ B. Canned goods

_____ C. Coffee, tea, other drinks or drink mixes

_____ D. Nuts, seeds

_____ E. Noodles, grains, rice, beans

_____ F. Baked goods, baking ingredients

_____ G. Vegetables, fruits

_____ H. Flavored mixes, such as gravy powder or packaged chili mix

_____ I. Seasonings, such as herbs, spices, vinegar, soy sauce, or salt

_____ J. Oil, lard, or vegetable shortening

7. The question that usually stops all self-deception: if the world suddenly suffered a shortage of pet food, would I be willing to feed my pet for a week from my own cupboard with complete confidence that the food would sustain the health and well-being of my beloved friend?

How your cupboards rate:

1. If you answered TRUE, you are stocking more processed food than fresh food. Fresh food has to be stored in the refrigerator. Many processed foods can be stored anywhere for an alarming length of time. To make the point, remember that World War II rations are still edible. If it's true that we are what we eat, you want to eat as much fresh food as possible. Limit the processed foods for embellishments or special treats.

2. If you answered TRUE, be advised that food over four months old is a clear indicator that you are not planning menus or budgeting your money well. Although many processed foods are perfectly good well beyond four months, there are better choices for you to make and better ways to manage your money than to spend it and park your investment on a shelf.

3. If you answered TRUE, you're a collector of food. One friend of ours defends this practice of buying and losing food as a great adventure of discovery. He enjoys the surprise of finding lost food as he digs around the kitchen for supper. He admits to feeling the triumph of a successful archaeologist when he unearths and opens an ancient tin to discover something (almost) edible (although suspicious). If you really enjoy this sort of adventure in culinary archeology, we encourage you to recognize it as recreation and limit it. There are better ways to nourish your body with fuel. Frankly, you need to learn to let go.

4. If you answered TRUE, then we have some work to do with you. Clearly, you have been more comfortable with canned and processed foods than with fresh foods. We frequently find that this preference develops because a person is busy, or interested in other things, or intimidated by cooking. Bad news: there is very little fuel in a can. Good news: It's easy to develop proficiency and efficiency in preparing fresh foods. Even better news: you can still have your canned food, but from now on you'll be using it to enhance a fresh meal.

5. If you answered TRUE, we rejoice to inform you that a talented, adventuresome athlete prepares the best meals. We regret to inform you that the

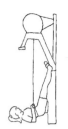

athlete who needs to embellish or mask natural flavors is a person seriously wedded to the idea that food must be delicious to be acceptable. (Before you get your knickers in a twist, we know you're not that weak and obsessed.) Our relationship with food is highly complicated. It's no secret that food satisfies many needs of the human spirit. But an athlete *must* distinguish emotional and spiritual needs from physical needs. Food is fuel. No more. No less. Decisions have to be made with logic and discipline. And the food you choose might not taste all that great if you are used to cookies and chips. You have to learn to sometimes trade delicious for nutritious, although the two are certainly not mutually exclusive.

6. Rank the following clusters of foods you have stored in your cupboard. A rank of one (1) means that you have more of this than anything else. A rank of ten (10) means that you have little or none of this.

A. Edibles in cellophane or plastic bags, such as packaged chips

High rank: You are attracted to snack foods. Likely you're a busy person and a little pressured. The vibrations generated as you munch a crunchy food release chemicals in the brain that calm and relieve tension. No wonder you enjoy them. Unfortunately, most snack foods are highly processed, and loaded with chemicals, fat, salt, and sugar. Additionally, they are intended to fill you up, but the calories tend to be empty. Cut back processed snack foods and become an expert label reader so you can replace them with nutritious alternatives. Now.

Low rank: You are a disciplined eater who does not eat solely for fun. Your priorities are in place. Good job.

B. Canned goods

High rank: You are either intimidated by preparing meals or you have been too busy in your life to spend time learning to cook. Canned goods, as we said earlier, are not the best source of regular nutrition for an athlete. Also, canned foods tend to be loaded with sugar, salt, and preservatives . . . lots of hidden calories and unexpected additives. Although you don't have to eliminate canned food, you need to limit its use and learn to enjoy fresh foods.

Low rank: You are an athlete who doesn't take shortcuts and who has learned to handle the kitchen and manage your meals along with your time. Your priorities are in place.

C. Coffee, tea, other drinks or drink mixes

High rank: Although there's not a lot wrong with coffee, tea, and other drinks, we have to issue a couple of warnings. Caffeine found in coffee, tea, cocoa, and some colas can be useful to an athlete; caffeine releases trans-fatty acids. Right before an event, this release can give you a little boost of energy. But caffeine is a natural diuretic and will dehydrate you if you ingest too much. Additionally, many commercial drinks contain sugar or sweeteners, which you don't need. The biggest objection we have to "drinks" is that while you're drinking one, you're not drinking water. If, as an athlete, you feel thirsty, your body is saying, "I need water." It's not saying, "I need iced tea." Granted, iced tea has water in it, and drinking tea will certainly satisfy your thirst. But not as well, not as purely, not as completely as water. Listen to your body.

Low rank: Good for you. You've learned to pour yourself a glass of water when you're thirsty. You've also acknowledged that no amount of caffeine can replace sleep when the body needs to be recharged, and no amount of sugar can replace energy when the body is exhausted.

D. Nuts, seeds

High rank: Bravo. In limited amounts, nuts and seeds are considered to be nature's finest snack foods. Watch out for seasonings, salts, and oils.

Low rank: There was nothing wrong with passing on nuts and seeds, but you might want to taste-test a few now. If you've relied heavily on packaged snack foods in the past, you might enjoy discovering nuts and seeds. They'll satisfy your need for "crunch." Additionally, their nutritional value is so high that you might want to experiment with putting them into, or sprinkling them on top of, other foods. By the way, we've had many athletes remark that nuts and seeds are good for dieting. It's impossible to lapse into mindless eating when you buy them in their shells and hulls. You'll have to work on each one in order to release the edible reward inside. We're not sure we can get too excited about the additional calories you'll burn as you shell, but we can guarantee that you'll slow down.

E. Noodles, grains, rice, beans

High rank: If you are using these as "extenders" in moderation, good for you. In order of preference, we rank brown rice first, beans second, whole grains third, and processed noodles fourth. Remember to try and eat foods that are as close to their natural state as possible.

Low rank: There's nothing wrong with limiting your intake of these carbohydrates, but you'll want to include them (even if only in small quantities) for energy in endurance activities.

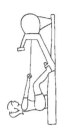

F. Baked goods, baking ingredients

High rank: It's hard to determine whether a high rank on baked goods is a positive or a negative influence on your nutritional profile. If you're addicted to grocery-store white bread and boxes of cookies, then you're in trouble. If you enjoy a daily serving of whole grain muffins you bake yourself, then you've done well. The continuum here is vast. All we can tell you is that you need to be careful in dealing with baked goods. Make sure your choices are good ones, and use discipline.

Low rank: There is nothing wrong with limiting baked goods. In fact, we would applaud eliminating all the empty calories, sugar, and salt loaded into cookies, cakes, and pastries. But there's something criminal about walking away from the niceties of our culture. We preach moderation in all things. You can live without baked goods, but why would you?

G. Vegetables, fruits

High rank: You've chosen well, Grasshopper. We favor vegetables and place them at the top of the menu at Wharton meals. Two important points: make sure your vegetables are fresh when you buy them, and buy vegetables in season. We use fruit more sparingly because of the sugar content, but we enjoy it every day as a treat. As with vegetables, we buy our fruit fresh and in season.

Low rank: No one ever admits to hating fruit, so we won't go there. But if you decided to rank vegetables low, we need to have a talk. Frankly, we cannot allow you to eliminate vegetables from your diet. In fact, we prefer that you not even limit your intake. We know there are some people who were traumatized by brussels sprouts when they were toddlers and haven't been near a vegetable since (exception: french fries). But it's time to get over it. The choices are vast. Surely we can find something you'll eat without gagging and running back to your brussels-sprouts-survivors' support group.

H. Flavored mixes, such as gravy powder or packaged chili mix

High rank: Caution is advised. Although these mixes are the saviors of busy cooks who want a fancy (effortless) dish on the table, they are loaded with empty calories, chemicals, fats, sugars, and salts. We aren't saying that they're all bad, we're just advising you to read the labels carefully and make informed choices.

Low rank: Good for you. Either you're an imaginative gourmet who wouldn't lower himself to relying on (perish the thought) packaged mixes, or you're a purist who has learned to enjoy simple foods. Either way, there's no need for you to concern yourself with these mixes.

I. Seasonings, such as herbs, spices, lemon juice, vinegar, soy sauce, or salt

High rank: We applaud the creative cook who can juice up a flavor with kitchen alchemy. We also enjoy the fact that when you do it yourself, you *know* what's going into the dish. No surprises in simple seasonings. But watch out for the high sodium content in soy sauce and many prepared seasonings. A little bit goes a long way.

Low rank: You might want to begin experimentation. As you learn to eliminate foods and embellishments high in fat, salt, and sugar, you might become bored with simple food. A little adventure with flavors can add excitement to your meals.

J. Oil, lard, or vegetable shortening

High rank: We do not disapprove of greasing the skids on a great dinner, but we have a huge problem if any of these (especially the lard) figure prominently in your kitchen. As always, we advise moderation in all things. And without question, not all oils are created equal. Choose wisely. We favor olive oil and canola oil (not lard) because they're monounsaturated.

Low rank: Good for you. You need a little oil in your diet, but you don't need a lot. Because fat occurs naturally in many foods, we are certain that you never need to add it (especially lard) to your diet.

7. Would you feel okay about imposing your diet on your pet for a week? If you answered yes, good for you. If you answered no, you need to rethink

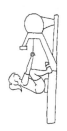

your diet. Of course we acknowledge that the dietary needs of humans and animals are different, but we are sometimes more conscientious about our pets than we are ourselves. For this reason, pets can serve as cornerstones of conscience and responsibility. This use of pets to evaluate one's diet came up one evening when we were at a party in the home of a friend. Our hostess was drinking a beer and eating from a small plate of fried cheese dipped in salsa. Her dog sat attentively beside her chair with his head on her lap, begging. Clearly, he wanted a nibble of dipped fried cheese and a dribble of her beer. She apologized to him, telling him, "No, sweetie. This isn't good for you. In fact, it would tear your stomach to shreds. You would be one unhappy puppy in the morning." Then she smiled lovingly and resumed her private little feast while her dog (who had apparently just been spared certain death) trotted away.

Jim and I looked at each other in disbelief. She had just acknowledged that her food and drink were just this side of lethal, and yet she still ate and drank. Jim couldn't help pointing out the irony: "Pal of mine, if you truly believe that this stuff is so terrible that you wouldn't feed it to your dog, why are you eating and drinking it?" There were a few seconds of icy silence (while a choice was being made between recognizing a moment of truth and pitching a full-blown temper tantrum). Then she said, "You're right. What am I thinking?" The snack went into the compost bin (where the dog probably sniffed it out later). The point is that if you wouldn't feed it to your dog, you shouldn't be eating it either. Sometimes we make better decisions when they are in regard to loved ones. It's a simple matter of recognizing that you, too, are a loved one in your own life. You deserve the best.

NOW THAT YOU KNOW HOW YOU EAT AND WHAT YOUR ATTITUDES ARE ABOUT FOOD, WE CAN PLAN

Let's review the five simple suggestions.

1. Make certain that 99 percent of what you eat is *food.*

You now know the difference between food and an edible. Make certain that you slow down your eating long enough to grasp the distinction between the two. Food is fuel; edibles are entertainment. You need the fuel. Edibles are packing empty calories, and wasting your time and money. They have a place, of course, in the pleasures of life. But their place is now limited.

2. Cut down sugar.

Cutting down on your sugar intake is simple. If it's sweet, it has sugar in it and you need to limit its intake. We're not telling you that you'll never have a candy bar again or that oranges are evil. We're merely suggesting moderation. And if you must have sugar, and can make a choice between fruit (a food) and processed sugar (an edible), please choose the food. Food is fuel.

3. Increase fiber.

A fiber-rich diet promotes healthy digestion and may be related to lower rates of colon cancer. It comes in two forms—soluble and insoluble. Insoluble fiber, found primarily in whole grains, fruits, and vegetables, provides bulk for the formation of stools and helps move wastes more quickly through the colon. Soluble fiber, found in peas and beans, many vegetables and fruits, and rice, corn, and oat bran, has been linked to lowering blood cholesterol levels. Good ways to get fiber into your diet are to eat fruit, add cooked beans and peas to soups and salads, use whole wheat flour whenever possible, eat whole grain foods, use brown rice instead of white, eat bran muffins instead of plain, and snack on fruits and vegetables.

4. Cut down fat.

The best way to cut down on fat is to invest in a calculator and become an avid reader of food labels. Use the information on the labels to keep your fat grams under 30 percent of the total calories you consume in a day. Then it's a simple matter of replacing fatty foods with less fatty foods. Let's assume that you perform best by consuming 2,200 calories a day. Following this general guideline, you calculate 30 percent of the 2,200 calories and set your goal: "I will consume no more than 660 calories of fat a day." There are 9 calories in a gram of fat. Dividing those calories by nine will tell you that you should eat no more than approximately 73 grams of fat.

A study at Pennsylvania State University identified techniques that were effective in achieving a diet with less than 30 percent of total calories from total fat. Because higher-fat meats and whole milk are the sources for a large percentage of fat in the American diet, the researchers targeted these foods for replacement with lower-fat substitutes. They discovered that simple, modest changes were easier for their research-dieters to handle, and more effective in achieving dietary goals than asking them to totally give up chips, cookies, and occasional treats. The work demonstrated that when you decrease fat in the diet, you automatically decrease calories. Although the goal is to become more healthy, a side benefit is weight loss. A person can lose between one half and one pound per week just by decreasing fat from 36 percent of calories to the recommended level of 30 percent. Even women in the study, because they had low calorie intake requirements and each food choice represented a larger proportion of the diet, lost weight most effectively by using combinations of simple changes that included replacing whole milk with skim milk, replacing high-fat meats with lean meats, and replacing full-fat products with fat-modified products.

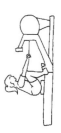

The Penn State researchers stressed that "by making simple changes, men and women can meet dietary goals for both total fat and saturated fat without depriving themselves of some of the higher-fat foods they enjoy." This position is supported by the new USFDA food guidelines, which suggest that we go easy on sugary drinks and treats, and cut down on meat, dairy products, and other sources of saturated fat.

CALORIES COUNT

Don't interpret "low-fat" and "fat-free" as a license to eat as much as you want. We have a friend who stuck to the percentage guidelines, quickly balancing his fat intake by eating low-fat bread. If he got too much fat in one day, he simply ate more bread . . . sometimes by the loaf. As long as the total intake of fat was under 30 percent, he felt righteous. He also felt his waistline expanding exponentially. It didn't take long for him to figure out that the point was to cut back fat, not increase everything else to hold the percentage in check.

Calories count, but be careful not to go too low. The fewer the calories, the more difficult it is to meet your daily requirements for nutrients to maintain good health.

5. Drink water.

Water is an important part of every healthy diet, but your requirements as an athlete are enormous. (You *are* sweating, aren't you? Good! We thought so.) Drinking eight to ten large glasses of water a day will help avoid dehydration. If you wish, you might use sports drinks designed especially for athletes. They're made to replace not only fluid, but sugars, salts, minerals, and electrolytes. Be aware of their contents and their calories. Staying adequately hydrated will also assist digestion and kidney function, and help control constipation. By the way, there is evidence that cold drinks are absorbed into the system more quickly than warmer ones. But use good judgment. If you're hot, drink cold water. But if you're cold, drink water that's warm or at room temperature.

"FAT-FREE" AND OTHER MYTHS

Until a couple of years ago, American consumers had to interpret food labels written by advertising copywriters, not nutrition experts. Information was confusing and often inaccurate. Today, the Food and Drug Administration and the U.S. Department of Agriculture and Inspection Service have standardized and regulated the language used. Now, a label says what it means and means what it says. That label is on the back of the package.

But many of us make a purchase selection based on the front of the package, where flash and promise play tricks on our logic. We think we are making an intelligent choice. Instead we make a mistake. It might be deceptive and it's certainly confusing, but it's all perfectly legal. It's up to you to understand what you've got in your shopping cart. Here are a few examples of descriptive verbiage and translations you can count on:

FAT

Fat-free: less than 0.5 grams of fat per serving

Saturated fat-free: less than 0.5 grams per serving and the level of trans-fatty acids does not exceed 1 percent of total fat

Low-fat: 3 grams or less per serving, and if the serving is 30 grams or less or 2 tablespoons or less, per 50 grams of the food

Low saturated fat: 1 gram or less per serving and not more than 15 percent of calories from saturated fatty acids

Reduced or less fat: at least 25 percent less per serving than reference food

Reduced or less saturated fat: at least 25 percent less per serving than the reference

CHOLESTEROL

Cholesterol-free: less than 2 milligrams of cholesterol and 2 grams or less of saturated fat per serving

Low-cholesterol: 20 milligrams or less and 2 grams or less of saturated fat per serving and, if the serving is 30 grams or less or 2 tablespoons or less, per 50 grams of the food

Reduced or less cholesterol: at least 25 percent less and 2 grams or less of saturated fat per serving than reference food

SUGAR

Sugar-free: less than 0.5 grams per serving

No added sugar, without sugar, or no sugar added: no sugars added during processing or packing (this includes ingredients that already contain sugar such as fruit juice); processing does not increase the sugar content above the amount naturally present in the ingredients

The food that it resembles and for which it substitutes normally contains added sugars.

If the food doesn't meet the requirements for a low- or reduced-calorie food, the product bears a statement that the food is not low-calorie or calorie-reduced and directs consumers' attention to the nutritional panel for further information.

Reduced sugar: at least 25 percent less sugar per serving than reference food

Low-calorie: 40 calories or less per serving, and if the serving is 30 grams or less or 2 tablespoons or less, per 50 grams of the food

Reduced or fewer calories: at least 25 percent fewer calories per serving than reference food

SODIUM

Sodium-free: less than 5 milligrams per serving

Low-sodium: 140 milligrams or less per serving and, if the serving is 30 grams or less or 2 tablespoons or less, per 50 grams of the food

Very low sodium: 35 milligrams or less per serving and, if the serving is 30 grams or less or 2 tablespoons or less, per 50 grams of the food

Reduced or less sodium: at least 25 percent less per serving than the reference food

FIBER

High-fiber: 5 grams or more per serving (By the way, foods making the high-fiber claim must meet the definition for low fat, or the level of total fat must appear next to the high-fiber claim.)

Good source of fiber: 2.5 grams to 4.9 grams per serving

More or added fiber: at least 2.5 grams more per serving than reference food

Also be aware that in athletic performance, if you feel thirsty, you're already dehydrated. It's a bad move and one certain to trash your workout, if not endanger your life. Drink before you need to.

In developing the discipline of drinking water, please don't leave your calculations to chance. Fill a bottle, or bottles, with your day's water supply and make sure you've drained it all before you go to bed. Drink intermittently throughout the day. Drink right before your workout, during your workout, and immediately following your workout. If you've drained your containers and still want more water, by all means, drink more.

We are frequently asked if other liquids besides water will do the job. The answer is yes, but not quite as well. Your body wants water. It's that simple. If you must drink other things, do so in addition to the water.

Go ahead and drink coffee and tea, but please practice moderation. Caffeine is a powerful central nervous system stimulant found in hundreds of foods (like chocolate), beverages, and drugs. And although you may now use it to feel more alert, there are compelling reasons that you should consider cutting back. Caffeine interferes with calcium absorption, and you need a positive balance in calcium to guard against osteoporosis. In addition, caffeine acts as a diuretic and may overload the bladder with urine, triggering or exacerbating urinary incontinence (loss of bladder control). For women in postmenopausal and later years, hot flashes and other uncomfortable symptoms may interfere with sleep. Caffeine makes falling asleep more difficult, decreases the time you stay asleep, and diminishes the quality of your sleep. To cut down, switch to decaffeinated versions of your favorite beverages. If you are a heavy drinker of caffeine and you quit cold turkey, you can expect some withdrawal symptoms such as irritability, nervousness, restlessness, lethargy, nausea, and headaches. Get tough and hang in there! They're temporary. To lessen any symptoms of withdrawal, cut back gradually.

Now that we've told you to cut it back, let us tell you about one instance when you might want to consider pouring it on. Caffeine frees fatty acids in the blood and makes energy available to fuel an endurance workout. Many marathon runners and long-distance cyclists will down a cup of coffee right before a workout to get an extra "edge." The actual benefits of this are a little controversial, but you might want to try it and see if it makes a difference in your performance. If it works at all, we would think that it would work more effectively if your overall caffeine levels are low—so we're still advising you to cut back on or eliminate caffeine from your diet.

FREE RADICALS AND ANTIOXIDANTS

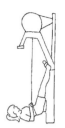

Just when you're feeling pretty good about getting a handle on your diet, we must inform you that every cell in your body is under a silent attack by a band of marauding renegades called free radicals. These are volatile, unstable oxygen molecules that career through your system and crash into other cells so hard that they actually produce sparks on impact. Why this wildly erratic and violent behavior? Free radicals have one or more unpaired electrons that demand pairing. Sometimes this pairing behavior is beneficial to you. Free radicals, when they're working properly and are in balance in your system, help you fight inflammation and infection, and help keep tone in the muscles of your internal organs and blood vessels. But all too often, the balance is disturbed between the free radicals doing a good job and the free radicals bent on destruction. The free radicals are made more powerful by air pollution, cigarette smoke, sunlight, environmental contaminants, and even too-much-too-soon exercise that damages fatigued cells. When the free radicals get out of control, they attack and can overwhelm healthy cells. Researchers are just beginning to understand the full impact of their destruction. Free radicals are now linked to cancers, cardiovascular disease, cholesterol elevation, cataracts, asthma, pancreatitis, inflammatory bowel diseases, Parkinson's disease, sickle-cell disease, leukemia, hypertension, rheumatoid arthritis, and many of the symptoms of premature aging. The list is terrifying . . . and growing.

The good news is that your body doesn't just stand by passively and let it happen. It marshals its troops. When your body detects too many renegade free radicals, it manufactures scavengers—endogenous antioxidants, whose mission is to seek out and destroy the renegades to keep them from doing any or further damage. It's a dramatic, classic Good vs. Evil power struggle, and one you can't afford to lose.

There are things you can do to help out the endogenous antioxidants that your body manufactures to defend your cells. You can eat a diet high in antioxidants—choose yellow, orange, and red fruits and vegetables and the "cruciferous" vegetables (broccoli, cauliflower, brussels sprouts)—and take antioxidant supplements—vitamins known to combat free radicals:

Vitamin C

Vitamin E

Beta-carotene

Check with your physician to confirm dosages and make sure it's safe for you to take these vitamins, but a general guideline is to take 400 IU of vitamin E,

1,000 mg of vitamin C, and 25,000 IU of beta-carotene. Additionally, you might check into the antioxidant multivitamins that combine everything into one formula. Again, we insist that you clear taking these supplements with your physician. Each supplement has side effects that are potentially harmful to certain people.

A WORD ABOUT WEIGHT LOSS

Although we have pointedly avoided the subject of weight loss in this chapter, no discussion of diet would be complete without a few remarks.

How Much Should You Weigh?

Of course, there are general guidelines, but everyone is a little different and the ranges can vary from person to person. How much you weigh seems to be less important than your total body composition and how much fat you carry. After all, your total weight reflects a composite of tissue, organs, skeleton, water, and clothing. Traditional strategies for assuring a more pleasing result from weighing yourself are to take off your shoes or urinate before you step onto the scale. In fact, we've seen desperate people cut their fingernails, take off jewelry, strip naked, and actually stand on tiptoe! These tricks may fool the scale into registering a lighter you, but the simple truth is that your fat content will not change. You are what you are. If you insist on weighing, see page 34.

Far more important is your ratio of fat to lean tissue, or your body composition. Determining your body composition will take the assistance of a health-care professional using skin-fold calipers or one of the high-tech electronic measuring devices, but you can get a general idea about whether you are fat (at risk) or lean (less at risk) by calculating your body mass index (BMI), a ratio between your height and weight, a formula that correlates with body fat.

(**Step 1**) Multiply your weight in pounds by 703.

(**Step 2**) Multiply your height in inches by your height in inches.

(**Step 3**) Divide the answer in Step 1 by the answer in Step 2 to get your BMI.

(**Step 4**) Round off that number.

Here's an example of how it would work for a person 5'5" tall and weighing 149 pounds:

(**Step 1**) Multiply your weight in pounds by 703. $149 \times 703 = 104{,}747$

(**Step 2**) Multiply your height in inches by your height in inches $65'' \times 65'' = 4{,}225$

(Step 3) Divide the answer in Step 1 by the answer in Step 2 to get your BMI. 104,747 ÷ 4,225 = 24.8

(Step 4) Round off that number. The person's BMI is 25.

Here's what your calculated BMI means:

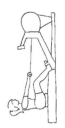

BMI CATEGORY	HEALTH RISK BASED ON BMI
Less than 25	Minimal
25 – < 27	Low
27 – < 30	Moderate
30 – < 35	High
35 – < 40	Very high
More than 40	Extremely high

So how do you get down to your ideal body mass index if you're carrying too much body fat right now? Follow our suggestions for healthy eating and then shave off a few calories from each meal. If you eat a healthy, balanced, moderately proportioned diet of real food, you're going to feel better immediately. As you feel better, you'll have more energy and be able to do more. As you do more, you'll burn more calories. As you burn more calories, you'll lose weight. As you lose weight, you'll be able to do even more. As you do even more, your muscle mass increases, and your body becomes more efficient at burning calories. You'll get leaner. It's that simple.

If you're worried about the discipline required in your diet, forget it. We have a wonderful surprise for you. As you begin your workouts, you'll suddenly discover a subtle shift in your relationship to your body. You'll notice small improvements in performance or time. As you start to get excited, you'll want to turn those small improvements into big ones. Suddenly, you'll be attracted to high-quality meals and be repelled by empty calories that would impede your progress. This attitude shift is a wonderful, natural, nearly effortless evolution in your maturity as an athlete. This is why the most effective weight/fat-loss programs are a combination of diet and exercise.

TAKE CHARGE NOW

Healthy diet and a healthy life go hand in hand, especially for an athlete. Making intelligent choices and mapping out an intelligent strategy for food selection, preparation, and consumption give you some effective controls over your well-being. Taking charge of your body often begins with taking charge of your grocery list.

> ## FINDING A QUALIFIED DIETITIAN
> If you have a hard time making changes in your diet, you might consider working with a registered, licensed dietitian, a health-care professional trained and uniquely qualified to work in concert with your physician to conduct an evaluation of your present medical status, help you set goals, and assist in planning and implementation of your new eating plan. You'll want to select one who specializes in *sports nutrition*. To find a dietitian, ask your physician for a referral, contact a local university nutrition department, look in the phone book, or explore the listing on the American Dietetic Association website at http://www.eatright.org.

13.
The Heart of a Woman

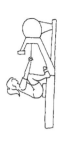

Our friend Caroline is a forty-six-year-old forest ranger in Idaho whose phone calls have always been exciting updates on her life in a log cabin and work in the mountains. Tales of her wilderness adventures and misadventures never failed to thrill the two of us, who live in an apartment in Manhattan and regard Central Park as the "great outdoors." About a year ago, Caroline placed a very different sort of call. She phoned to let us know that she was in the hospital after having suffered a heart attack. We thought she was kidding. When we expressed disbelief, she assured us that we could not be more shocked than she was. After all, she was a young, active woman. Heart attacks, we three agreed, appeared to have been the exclusive domain of men. Weren't they? Caroline said sadly, "All my life, I maintained that I was equal to men. Frankly, this isn't what I had in mind."

Caroline's heart attack might have been equal opportunity—without respect for her gender—but the story of her symptoms, diagnosis, and treatment were quintessentially female. She had suffered chest pain earlier in the day, but casually passed it off as a touch of indigestion. When antacids failed to soothe away the problem, Caroline had become mildly concerned. As the hours passed, she felt increasing pressure in her chest and experienced nausea. Although she scanned her experience for an explanation, at no point had she considered the possibility of a heart attack. Six hours after the onset of symptoms, she drove herself to her physician, who listened to Caroline's complaints, examined her briefly, and attempted to reassure our scared friend with his best "calm down and you'll be all right and stay away from that curry next time" speech. He prescribed a stronger antacid. Caroline collapsed in the hallway outside his office door.

Before you conclude that Caroline is an idiot, and her physician should be strangled with his own stethoscope, let us tell you that they *both* behaved predictably. Dealing with heart problems is the one arena in medicine where gender differences and cultural biases play important and deadly roles. When a man experiences chest pain, the first thing he thinks is, "Heart attack!" If he presents even one of Caroline's symptoms to his physician, the physician thinks, "Heart attack!" Not so with the female patient and her physician, neither of whom is likely to jump to that conclusion. In fact, heart disease is more difficult to diagnose through tests in women than men, even when the physician suspects it's the culprit. Fortunately, Caroline's case had a happy outcome (she's doing great!), but many women don't survive the litany of misconceptions and misinformation that have been the signatures of women's coronary health care in the past. The good news is that survival rates are improving as women become better educated, heart studies include more women, diagnostic tools become more sophisticated, and the medical community becomes better informed.

CORONARY ARTERY DISEASE

Most heart attacks are caused by coronary artery disease. The disease strikes when a coronary artery—a large vessel that feeds blood to the heart—becomes clogged with hard plaque. When blood can't get through to the heart to deliver nutrients and oxygen, the heart muscle suffers damage. Cardiovascular disease is the leading cause of death of both men and women in the United States. More than 250,000 women die from heart attacks every year and another 250,000 die from other cardiovascular diseases. (To put this statistic into perspective, 46,000 women die of breast cancer each year.)

Heart attack is only one of the possible outcomes of untreated cardiovascular disease. We started our discussion with the heart attack because of our friend Caroline's frightening diagnosis, and because it is one of the most visible manifestations of cardiovascular disease. Among the others are angina—chest pain signaling that the heart muscle is not receiving enough oxygen, and silent ischemia—a dangerous, symptomless, painless reduction in blood flow to the heart. By the way, silent ischemia frequently goes undiagnosed in women who do not insist on cardiac testing during their physical exams. Without early detection, diagnosis might come when it is too late.

Another frightening manifestation of cardiovascular disease is high blood pressure—hypertension. Half of all diagnosed hypertensive patients are women, and they surpass their male counterparts statistically after age forty-five. Hypertension causes constriction in blood vessels that should be pumping blood through the body. As blood flow becomes more constricted and less efficient, the vessels work harder to compensate, and are strained and damaged. Organs that count on blood flow for oxygen and nutrients, and no longer get what they need, begin to fail. Hypertension, if untreated, can lead to heart failure, renal damage, and stroke. Stroke, one of the most insidious killers associated with cardiovascular disease, is the third leading cause of death. Statistics indicate that although more men than women suffer stroke, women are more likely to die from the event. Simply put, when the brain doesn't get blood flow, cells begin to die within minutes, gradually and systematically shutting down all the mental and physical functions governed by the brain cells being starved: in lay terms, a stroke. The results range widely from a temporary loss of function to death.

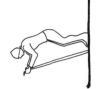

MEN AND WOMEN ARE DIFFERENT

What do we know about the differences between men and women with regard to cardiovascular disease? While it's true that men's and women's hearts are anatomically identical, women are smaller than men, and so are their hearts and arteries. So it takes less plaque to clog an artery and shut off blood flow in a woman's smaller heart. Additionally, women enjoy the apparent cardioprotective effects of estrogen until menopause (sometime in midlife), and therefore tend to be older than their male counterparts when first diagnosed with heart disease. The disease might have progressed further by the time it's discovered and be only one of a litany of health problems associated with advancing age, and therefore harder to diagnose and treat.

Another surprising difference between men and women is that our culture today puts more stress on women, who struggle to balance unrelenting family responsibilities against the demands of career. Unlike the traditional male role in our society, where Papa comes home from a hard day's work and kicks back to relax, studies indicate that Mama comes home from that same day's hard work and still launches into an evening of household chores, carting kids to soccer practice, whipping up supper, supervising homework, and helping care for aging parents. Statistics tell us that some women have exacerbated the physically disabling problems of pressure by turning to alcohol, smoking, and substance abuse—refuges for relaxation (of the worst sort). To be certain, the world is changing to level the homefront workload, but not quickly enough to shelter women from pressure right now. In fact, statistics show that the death rate from cardiovascular disease has fallen more rapidly for men than women over the past twenty years. However, we are experiencing a societal shift in men's and women's roles that hopefully will ease the pressure on women. We also look forward to more research results, and better diagnosis and treatment for women's cardiovascular disease.

So where did we ever get the idea that women are not candidates for cardiovascular disease? Some researchers have identified the female hormone estrogen as being a shield between women and cardiovascular disease. Much of the information we have about estrogen's cardioprotective nature comes from studies done on oral contraceptives (birth control pills), estrogen replacement therapy in postmenopausal women whose ovaries no longer produce the hormone, and the effects of menopause (natural and surgically induced) on women's risk of heart disease. However, recent studies of the benefits of postmenopausal hormones are equivocal. We now know that after menopause, when estrogen levels decline, total cholesterol levels rise an average of 25 points, increasing the risk of developing heart disease by 50 percent. However, when a woman takes oral estrogens to replace her declining levels, LDL cholesterol (the "bad" kind) drops and HDL cholesterol (the "good" kind) increases. Additionally, some studies indicate that postmenopausal replacement estrogens slightly lower blood pressure. Estrogen is believed to decrease the stickiness of platelets, a phenomenon that causes blood cells to adhere to one another and to form dangerous clots. Clotting is nature's way of stopping blood flow when a person is cut, but clots can form inside a blood vessel, sealing it off and causing a heart attack or stroke. Estrogen also stimulates the artery walls, causing the release of nitric oxide, which dilates or opens the arteries. At the same time, estrogen inhibits the release of endothelin, which constricts the arteries. Additionally, estrogen relaxes the smooth muscle tissue beneath the lining of the artery. The net effect is increased blood flow, which helps a healthy heart. Estrogen also appears to protect the lining of the blood vessel walls, where plaque forms and shuts off blood flow. Studies indicate that estrogen users have less narrowing than nonusers, even in the presence of other cardiovascular risk factors such as high blood pressure, cigarette smoking, diabetes, and obesity. In fact, some studies indicate that estrogens appear to reduce the risk of cardiovascular disease by up to 63 percent. Of course, not every woman is a candidate for estrogen replacement therapy. In fact, there are several compelling circumstances under which taking estrogen could be dangerous, such as when a patient has unexplained vaginal bleeding or breast, endometrial, or ovarian cancer. A woman's physician will be able to examine risk factors, and make a recommendation.

As research continues, we'll have more information regarding women, estrogen, and the prevention of cardiovascular disease, but until then, women of all ages, no matter where they are on the estrogen-level continuum, should remain vigilant against disease and guard their health as conscientiously as men. This requires planning and sticking to intelligent diet and exercise programs. Research strongly suggests that the relationship between excess body weight and cardiovascular disease may be stronger in women than in men. Even a few extra pounds appear to increase the risk dramatically. If you smoke, quit immediately. If you drink alcohol, do so in moderation. Get your cholesterol under control, and keep it there. And get regular physical checkups that include cardiac testing.

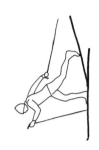

Cardiovascular disease is an equal-opportunity killer without respect for gender. Women, like men, deserve a lifetime of glowing good health, so it is important to take charge today.

14.
Fitness Is Child's Play

Our neighbor Karen Sorenson cornered us in the hall by the elevator one morning, where she obviously had been waiting for us. Cordial greetings were cut short by her abrupt announcement that she needed a fitness program. She wanted to schedule a consultation in our clinic—the sooner the better. "Sure, Karen. We'd love to design a program for you!" She thrust a file folder into Phil's hands. She said, "It's not for me. It's for Joe. Here's the medical report. You'll see for yourselves. We have to do something fast or . . ." Her voice trailed off, and the unfinished explanation was punctuated by an ominous silence. Jim asked, "What's wrong?" Karen whispered, "He failed his physical fitness test. He's twenty-two percent above his ideal weight. You know that makes him technically obese. He has high blood pressure and his cholesterol's too high. The doctor said that we could get it all under control with exercise and diet. Can you help?" We said, "You've come to the right neighbors. Let's get on it. We'll review this file, and you bring Joe to the clinic after he gets off from work tonight." Karen was momentarily flustered. "Jim, Phil, I'm not talking about my husband Joe. I'm talking about my *son*, Joe Jr." Young Joe was nine years old. As shocking as the Sorensons' story is, it's a scenario being repeated across the country with alarming frequency. Frankly, there's no excuse for a generation of unhealthy, unfit children.

Fitness is child's play. Literally. For children to achieve or maintain fitness, all they have to do is open the front door and step out into the world of perpetual motion, boundless energy, and unbridled fun. Our culture today places a premium on recreation and leisure, so there's ample opportunity for children to participate in games and sports. Yet there's a terrible irony. Abysmal research results tell us that kids in the United States today are less fit than kids a generation ago. Test scores for distance running and general fitness have declined 10 percent in the past twenty years. Kids weigh more and have higher fat content than kids of their parents' generation. One out of five kids between the ages of six and seventeen is overweight. Forty percent of kids aged five to eight exhibit signs of early cardiovascular disease or have at least one heart disease risk factor (including elevated serum cholesterol levels, lowered cardioprotective high density lipoproteins, and high blood pressure). And these alarming childhood statistics are only the beginning. Unhealthy, unfit kids frequently grow up to be unhealthy, unfit adults. Indeed, strong evidence suggests that the foundation for adult health and fitness—good and bad—begins in childhood. Researchers suspect that some cardiovascular basics are laid in place early in life. And all agree that lifetime habits can be formed and firmly set in stone.

Something is going horribly wrong.

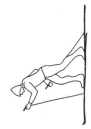

So what's the problem? Economic difficulties in public school systems are forcing cutbacks. Among the first programs to get the ax are physical fitness programs. In fact, the American Heart Association reports that less than 36 percent of elementary and secondary schools offer daily gym classes. There's more bad news. Even if a school offers a program, the curriculum isn't likely to include classes in fitness skills that can be sustained and enjoyed for a lifetime. Frustrated school administrators quickly point out that children are in school only a few hours a day, only five days a week, and that parents share responsibility for educating their kids—fitness included. Sure, it's a logical argument for a healthy balance between schoolwork and play, but the reality for many kids is that activity at home consists of planting themselves in front of the television set or computer screen. Studies indicate that kids sit and stare at a screen for an average of sixteen to twenty hours per week. And many parents don't mind. As long as Junior is watching TV or surfing the Internet, he's contentedly occupied, thoroughly entertained, and safe from the menacing outside world. Junior slowly evolves from being one of life's players into one of its spectators. And his gradual slide into inactivity takes an insidious lifelong toll on his health.

We would like to offer a simple solution: limit screen time. We stress moderation in most things, so we're not telling you to throw the circuit breaker forever. What we *are* saying is to choose wisely when directing children's time. Every minute that a child sits in front of a screen is one minute that he or she isn't running and jumping. Those minutes add up into idle hours, and those hours rob a kid of life.

By the way, limiting screen time is a wise strategy for *all* people, not just children. We once had an adult client who came to our clinic to be treated for carpal tunnel syndrome, developed from playing video games in his spare time. When we gently suggested that he get his duff off the couch occasionally and swap his joystick for a hockey stick, he informed us that playing video games provided a perfectly adequate cardiovascular workout. In fact, he could get his heart rate racing by piloting his on-screen Starflight Cruiser past the Wizard to do battle with the evil Lizard Masters (or something like that). And further, he huffed, no mere hockey player had ever personally saved the universe from complete annihilation. He was impressive, to be sure, but totally off the mark. Trust us. If the universe needs to be saved from evil Lizard Masters, we assure you that it's going to be done by physically fit, healthy people with energy, stamina, strength, coordination, and flexibility. And *none* of those people will have achieved all that by sitting in front of a screen.

Our collective societal slide into sloth—adults and children alike—is being greased by sitting in front of televisions and computer screens. The first step toward physical fitness is to limit screen time, and use those newly freed hours to engage in physical activity. Work out. Play. Enjoy the game of life.

PARENTS, PRACTICE "FOLLOW THE LEADER"— YOU LEAD

The single most important factor in encouraging a child's participation in physical activity is the parent. Whenever we have a discussion regarding the importance of the parent's function as a role model in order to nurture a fit child, Jim Wharton (the father and athlete) simply points to Phil Wharton (the son and athlete) and rests his case. Take it from a caring father: if you want healthy children, you have to be the leader, to show them the way, to set the example. Fitness is one aspect of life where action speaks louder than words. Inactive parents have no credibility when they nestle into the couch and resort to chanting the old adage "Do as I say and not as I do." The successful pursuit of fitness as a lifestyle is a joyful family affair. When your kitchen is stocked with healthy foods and the culture of your entire family is one that supports health, physical activity, and fitness together, kids are clear that it's fun. They grow up valuing health, physical activity, and fitness. Further, they develop good habits and interests that last a lifetime.

CHOOSING THE RIGHT ACTIVITY FOR CHILDREN

Unfortunately, adults use the term "work out" when describing a fitness program. We say "unfortunately" because the word "work" instantly invokes images of some unpleasant effort in return for reward. Adults, by nature, work at getting fit. (By the way, this misconception quickly evaporates as surprising and satisfying gains are made in health and fitness.) Children, on the other hand, never look at physical activity as work. On the contrary, to them, it's play.

Play is the foundation of fitness. Play fits nicely into four distinct categories or levels that become increasingly complex. Kids start with the first, and then as they mature, they increase participation to include the next level of activity. Please note that levels don't replace one another; they are merely added. Each remains an important component of the human experience, a fact that adults sometimes forget.

Level One: Simple noncompetitive activities

Examples: swinging and jumping rope

This is play without structure or rules. Kids can play alone, but because this is freewheeling, pets and other people can easily be included.

Level Two: Games

Examples: "Ring Around the Rosie" and "Swing the Statue"

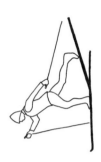

This play introduces structure and rules. If you've ever heard a kid say, "Hey, you're not doing it right!" then you know that play has progressed to games. Additionally, games are played with an expected result or outcome. Something is supposed to happen that will signal success and completion. Compare swinging (simple noncompetitive activity) with "Ring Around the Rosie" (game). When kids swing, they engage in the activity for the pleasure of it. The activity ends when the kids are tired of it. On the other hand, "Rosie" requires kids to memorize and sing a song, to hold hands and form a circle, to move in the same direction while keeping step to the song, and finally to fall on the ground on cue. Like simple noncompetitive activity, the game doesn't have competitors (winners or losers), but it does have an expected successful outcome—kids falling on the ground and doing it so well that they don't have to let go of one another's hands. When a kid begins to measure his or her ability to participate against that of the other kids, competition begins. The idea of performing better—winning—makes the game infinitely more interesting as a kid matures.

Level Three: Organized team sports

Examples: softball and soccer

Because most kids are first introduced to sports in school, their first foray onto the playing field is on teams. Kids develop strength, flexibility, coordination, balance, stamina, and skill using the sport as a context or a laboratory. This on-the-field development is like learning to play the piano: you can learn one skill at a time and then put them all together to finally play a song, but it's more fun to develop skills as you learn to play the song. Team sports are much the same. They require a complex amalgam of skills, best learned as kids play, and refined as they mature. Team sports also teach kids that when they organize and cooperate with other people, they can accomplish more as a group than they can individually. Each player brings his or her own special talents and skills to the effort, no one more or less important. In organized team sports, too, the concept of winning and losing is introduced for the first time. Kids learn that success sometimes means defeating an opponent. The activity is no longer for the sheer fun of it. Now there are stakes.

Level Four: Organized individual sports

Examples: singles tennis and handball

Individual sports are highly sophisticated competitions, the reason being that the athlete launches into a game unassisted by friends. No one will be there to fill in the gaps, to consult for strategy, to rely on when things get tough, or to blame when things get tougher. At this point, the game becomes a lesson in self-reliance—one warrior against another in a battle scenario as old as time. The child discovers that it's lonely at the top . . . and even lonelier at the bottom. Winning and losing become deeply personal. And life's lessons are invaluable.

By the way, these four levels of play come full circle in adulthood, when grown-ups often revert to simple play. Organizing teams and events into professional work schedules and busy lives is difficult. But the call to play is instinctive in us, so we find alternatives, recreation for one. Working out at the gym, running, cycling, swimming, or any of the activities like those in this book are simple play . . . almost. As adults, we can hardly resist the notion of outcome (and successful outcome at that!). We generally set a goal at the outset of the activity, and we refine the activity to meet that goal. But at the heart of the workout is simple play, just for the sheer fun of it.

WHAT PLAY TEACHES US

A joyful body in motion develops strength, flexibility, coordination, reflexes, cardiovascular capacity, and cognitive and motor skills. But play's benefits go far beyond the physical. Games and sports parody life, staging little comedies and dramas that are rehearsals for the real thing. Kids learn how the world works, how to solve problems, work with other people, cooperate, and understand strengths, limitations, and compensations. They learn when to lead and when to follow. They learn how to succeed and, equally important, how to fail. They learn how to dream big, then to handle a dream that becomes a nightmare. They learn how to be fair and how to cope with a world that's not. They learn how to be powerful, competent, and masterful, one step at a time. And, most of all, they learn how to have fun.

Play, with all its benefits, comes so naturally to children that we are tempted to advise parents to merely get out of the way, but, in fact, it's a parent's responsibility to guide. Not all play is created equal, and you want to be sure your child is developmentally ready to engage in an activity before you encourage participation. For example, your child might enjoy running, but marathon running is inappropriate for a small body. Your child might express interest in weight lifting, but competitive body building is inappropriate for a small body. How do you know which sports are appropriate? We first rely on common sense. You know your child's capabilities. If you take a look at the activity, interview the coach or teacher, and determine that there could be a successful match, then you might allow limited, supervised participation until you're certain that your child can handle it and will enjoy it. If in doubt, keep in mind that most sports have a governing body. Get in touch with the experts and ask their advice. All will give you their recommendations and guidelines for participation. And finally, we encourage you to select activities, sports, and games where you can play together.

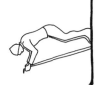

FAMILY FUN

Here are a few activities that will rev up heart rates and can be enjoyed by adults and children together. Note that all should be noncompetitive. We discourage activities within families that foster the concept of winners and losers. We think it's more productive if all the family members have fun together and support one another as a team—all on the same side. (Save the competitive stuff for later, more important issues like battles over car keys and bathrooms.)

Walking
Hiking
Dog walking
Climbing
Orienteering
Exploring with a camera or binoculars
Camping
Running
Scooter riding
Surfing
Bodysurfing

Swimming

Snorkeling

Waterskiing

Cycling

In-line skating

Skateboarding

Snow skiing

Snowboarding

Snow-fort building

Cross-country skiing

Snowman building

Ice skating

Sledding

Tobogganing

Gardening and yard work

Horseback riding

Carpentry

Pitching and catching a ball

Jumping rope

Rowing, canoeing, kayaking, and rafting

Stilt building and walking

Pogo-stick jumping

Frisbee tossing

Swinging and other playground activities

Dancing

Skipping

Kite flying

Playing hopscotch

Trampoline jumping

Golf putting

Somersaulting and tumbling on the lawn

KID-SIZED FATIGUE

When you take a young child out to play, he or she is in charge of having fun. You're in charge of everything else. It's up to you to keep in mind the differences in your size, strength, energy, and perceptions of time and distance. We learned an important lesson from friends who took their five-year-old daughter on a hike to explore the woods near their home in northern New York. The three were looking for a hidden mine shaft that was a favorite destination of local day-trippers in search of adventure. The parents knew that the mine was "just around the next bend," but the child grew weary and had difficulty with the concepts of "almost" and "any minute now" and "just a few more yards." For the parents, the hunt for the mine meant a walk in the woods for their family, drawn onward by delicious anticipation. For their daughter, it apparently meant a forced march through hell, marked by fatigue, frustration, disappointment, and mind-numbing boredom. Inevitably, she concluded that there was a fine line between an adult's idea of adventure and a five-year-old's idea of child abuse. She suggested they discuss their differences. (Well, actually she threw herself onto the ground and intelligently refused to take another tortured step.) Fortunately for our friends and their daughter, a short rest and a snack from the backpack restored peace. And even better, that mine *was* just around the next bend. Was the discovery worth the effort? Not if you're talking about finding the mine. But if you're talking about our friends becoming sensitive to the differences between tall parents and short daughters, you bet it was.

The point is that getting your child involved in fitness means that you, too, have to get involved. But when you organize family activities that include everyone, you have to keep your child in mind. Only when an activity's well suited to his or her capabilities and interests is it fun. And even though the activity might not challenge you fully, when something's fun for your child, it'll be fun for you. Trust us. When you play with your family, you're doing more than building healthy bodies and a foundation for lifelong fitness: you're building a strong family bond and wonderful memories. Enjoy.

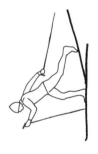

A WORD ABOUT DEHYDRATION AND KIDS

Children can become so absorbed in play that they forget to drink. Adequate hydration is important for all people, but might be especially so for children. Scientists warn us that the smaller the person, the greater the ratio of body surface area to body mass. This means that, relative to a fully grown adult, a child's body has more surface area through which to absorb heat. Additionally, a child's sweat glands produce only about 40 percent of the sweat they'll produce when they mature. Sweat is nature's coolant. As it evaporates off the skin, the body cools down. Because a child has a limited capacity to produce sweat, he or she can't cool as quickly as an adult. It's a double whammy that an active kid needs help managing. We suggest that all hard physical activity—especially in heat or humidity—be supervised by a vigilant adult with a large water bottle and the good sense to know when a kid needs to "cool it" and come inside. We advise all athletes to drink. Kids are no different.

By the way, we've had great success in hydrating our young athletes by supplying water or fluids in pop-top "squirt" bottles that can be purchased in any grocery or convenience store that stocks energy replacement drinks. Kids get a kick out of them. Although the price of the bottled product might seem outrageous, think of it as an investment. Long after your child has drained the expensive drink, the bottle can be refilled with more economical fluids—like water—and reused.

15.
Saving the Best for Last: The Older Athlete

Bad news. There is no Fountain of Youth. If there were, Ponce de León would still be among us. And as we all know, he aged gracefully and passed away a long time ago. (You *did* know that, didn't you?) Of course, we like to think that old Ponce's last years were wonderful ones . . . not because he was soaking wet and regressing to his childhood, but because he was in Florida, where the weather is warm and it's easier to stay active year-round. To be fair, Ponce de León was on the right track: getting wet *is* a key component in maintaining or regaining vigor. But it's not a matter of soaking in a fountain, it's a matter of generating sweat—getting your heart rate up with regular physical exercise.

One of the characteristics associated with aging is slowing down, but we want to issue a challenge to that perception. More and more research demonstrates that, to a great extent, slowing down might be the cause, not the effect, of some of the "symptoms" we formerly associated with aging. Of course, speeding up a body that's slowing down a little takes effort. Aging appears to coincide with a slow loss of muscle mass—about 1 percent per year after age thirty. Muscles are like furnaces that burn fat for energy. As muscle mass diminishes, the body can't burn fat as efficiently, becoming less lean and more fat. This combination forms a sort of vicious cycle. Less muscle means more fat means even less muscle, which means even more fat, which means . . . well, you get the picture. It's called "creeping atrophy" for good reason. It happens slowly, starting as early as our twenties. By the time a person notices that body parts are drifting, and anatomical peaks and valleys are becoming redistributed, the cycle has a firm hold on its victim. Unless checked, the consequences are debilitating and insidious. In the past, we accepted these declines as normal functions of aging, but not anymore. Now we're learning ways to break the cycle. Of course, the earlier you start, the better. But we know that it's never too late if one is relatively healthy and able to move. Studies demonstrate that older people can do very well and make remarkable progress in fitness, no matter

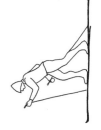

when they start. Research and experience have demonstrated that we can indeed stay well and healthy in our later years by engaging in a fitness program. In fact, exercise may be the best-kept antiaging secret around.

We had a sixty-five-year-old client working out in our clinic one afternoon when a well-intentioned (younger) person advised, "Take it easy. You're not as young as you used to be." We all laughed out loud. The older client could have bench-pressed the younger one and then jogged all the way to Brooklyn with that guy slung over his shoulder. It was a typical case of underestimating the capabilities of the older body, particularly the body of a man who had been working out for a while. We knew better. And now so does the younger man.

Baby boomers are changing the face of aging. They are plunging headlong into their later years, bringing with them a lifestyle that embraces health and fitness. The icons of retirement used to be shuffleboard and rocking chairs. Not anymore. Today we're more likely to associate retirement with more time to train for that marathon and travel to South America to run the rapids in a kayak. The myths are exploding. The limitations are being shoved back. In the battle against aging, the gloves are off. And the running shoes are on.

THE SPECIAL BENEFITS OF FITNESS FOR OLDER PEOPLE

Because physical inactivity is associated with many medical problems associated with aging, it stands to reason that getting fit will absolutely improve your health and might prolong your life.

You'll get a fresh outlook on life.

Studies tell us that cardiovascular exercise is one of the best antidotes for depression. The effects of exercise are grounded in both psychology and physiology. First, the more fit you become, the more control you take over your life. Health improves. You feel better. Fat begins to melt as your self-esteem builds. Your attitude improves and depression lifts. But the attitude isn't the only thing changing. There is a physiological basis for this lift. When you put your body through the stresses of prolonged exercise, your brain produces chemicals that calm you, deaden minor pain, change your perceptions of time and effort, and stimulate you to feel pleasure. Your body literally generates its own mood elevator. The effect lasts beyond the workout and is so compelling that you won't be able to wait to come back for more. (You've always wondered why athletes smile a little more than you thought they should. Now you know.)

You'll gain strength.

As we noted earlier, there is a slow loss of muscle mass as life progresses—about 1 percent per year after age thirty. As muscle mass diminishes, the body can't burn fat as efficiently, becoming less lean and more fat. This combination means that you might put on weight (fat) more quickly than you thought possible. Adding muscle mass means you increase your capacity to burn fat. The result is that you'll stay leaner longer. Additionally, a strong body works better structurally. You'll stand more erect. Your internal organs will be held in place more firmly so that they function properly. You'll be more capable physically for longer.

You'll be more balanced.

One of the most ridiculous stereotypes of older people is that they shuffle, dodder, and totter. Nonsense. Again we stress that physical limitations are not necessarily functions of aging. They are more likely the consequences of a lifetime of physical inactivity, resulting in weak muscles, inflexibility, dulled reflexes, and structural instability. Studies of men and women who maintain (or regain) even modest levels of fitness suggest that we can leave the idea of shuffling, doddering, and tottering at the door of the gym. There are good reasons to want to stay on your toes. When you hit a bump on the path, you need to be able to react quickly to regain equilibrium. If you're not strong or agile enough to catch yourself, you'll certainly hit the ground. If you suffer from some degree of osteoporosis, you can bet that porous bones are likely to break. If you're inflexible, you can count on strained, sprained, or torn connective tissues in a joint. A good way for us to illustrate the benefits of being in shape to prevent or minimize falls is to point out the way children deal with tumbles. Most of the time, they are able to catch themselves. If that fails, they're usually able to roll out of the fall, often in elaborate acrobatics that will result in a full recovery back to upright and a good laugh. We know you're thinking, "Yeah, but the bigger you are, the harder you fall." That's true. You can't change your height. But maybe that's even more reason for you to maintain fitness.

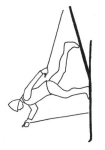

Your love life will improve.

With complete disregard for discretion and decorum, we are going to tell you that we know for a fact that sexuality is as important when we grow older as it is when we are younger. How do we know this? We study the research (and confidentially, we are two generations of Whartons—father and son—who can personally confirm the research). Why doesn't everyone know this? In our culture, much of what we think we know about one another is gathered from our exposure to media, and media focuses on the young. Consequently, those of us who are younger have no clue that romance extends beyond middle age. And those of us who are older get to be pleasantly surprised . . . unless we're unhealthy or unfit. For both males and females, as the body ages, there tends to be a degradation of the endocrine system and a reduction in the production of hormones that are important to the stimulation of libido, and to the physiology of making love itself. Exercise enhances the body's ability to produce those critical hormones, and keeps the fun in your love life.

Of course, it goes without saying that making love is a physical activity, made more enjoyable by being healthy, flexible, and fit. Also, we delicately mention that although it is rarely classified technically as an aerobic activity, it does get the heart rate up for a period of time. In spite of this, we cannot recommend making love as the basis of a fitness program. We do, however, point out that your athletic performance in all activities is enhanced by being in great shape.

You'll prevent or slow down osteoporosis.

Osteoporosis means "porous bones" and refers to the degenerative disease that results in severe bone loss. If you think that osteoporosis is a problem only for women, think again. While it's true that 80 percent of all victims of osteoporosis are women, men are at risk, too. From birth until early adulthood, bone is constantly replacing itself. At any given time, from 5 to 20 percent of your skeleton is rebuilding or remodeling itself. Then, at about age thirty-five, you reach your peak bone mass, and the dynamic process of rebuilding begins to slow down. At this point, bone loss exceeds production. Calcium absorption also declines, and your body's ability to manufacture vitamin D is diminished. In women, when menopause factors into the equation, and estrogen levels decline or drop completely, the body loses even more of its ability to absorb calcium (estrogen helped). The result is that a woman can lose up to 35 percent of her cortical bone mass (thin, dense bone that covers trabecular bone and is found in arms and legs) and 50 percent of her trabecular bone (latticework bone formation found primarily in the spine, breastbone, ends of long bones, and top of pelvis) over her lifetime. If bone loss is severe or continues over a long period, the bones become too fragile to withstand everyday physical stress, and they fracture. Unfortunately, osteoporosis in both women and men has no obvious early symptoms. A fracture may be the first signal that things are going wrong.

Before you pack yourself in Styrofoam peanuts, we have good news for you. Load-bearing exercise strengthens bones and slows down the effects of osteoporosis. Load-bearing means that you stress the muscles, connective tissues, and bones with weight. For example, swinging your arm from side to side is not load-bearing, but lifting a tennis racket is. So is walking, where your legs impact the ground, bear the weight of and support your body, and propel you forward. You get the idea. We have more good news for you: the exercise doesn't have to be strenuous to do you some good. In terms of load, more is not necessarily better. The idea is to get out there, and do it regularly and to the extent that you are able.

EXPECT RESULTS

The disabilities associated with aging develop slowly over a lifetime, so you can't expect to win a slot on the Olympic team within one month. But you can expect significant improvement in a very short period of time. In fact, many people feel better from the get-go. Almost everyone, no matter how sedentary, has secretly thought, "I need to get my duff into a program." It's as though we all have some sort of cellular memory of what it was like to be a kid who could jump on the bed and climb trees and skip down the sidewalk. Once that joyful, effortless movement is gone, there is a longing to get back to it. Somehow. Someday.

Well, somehow is with this book. And someday is *today.* There is great satisfaction in finally taking control, and in getting yourself off the couch and out the front door. At this moment, you are the least fit you will ever be again. It's over. From the first step you take, you have broken the sloth cycle. We have a nutritionist friend who advises his private clients that the first step toward successful weight loss is figuring out how to *not* gain any more weight. You need to throw on the brakes. Once you've conquered the weight gain, you can master the weight loss. The same is true of a return to fitness. Once you've conquered sloth, you can master fitness. It's a moment of decision. You decide, once and for all, that enough is enough. And it will be.

BEFORE YOU START YOUR FITNESS PROGRAM, CLEAR YOUR PLANS WITH YOUR PHYSICIAN

In fact, you might even check in with a sports-medicine physician or a cardiologist. Take this book with you and discuss the program that interests you. Make sure you can handle it, or have your physician make suggestions on modifying the program to suit you.

TIPS FOR STICKING TO YOUR PROGRAM

Let's be honest. It's tough to begin a new fitness program when you've been inactive your whole life. There are new skills to learn and old habits to break. You have to develop more discipline than you've ever had before. It's not easy, but it's critical. Once you decide you're going to get fit, get with the program.

Put your program together with realistic expectations. Take it slowly. Remember that you're *always* in full control. (This is one of the great secret pleasures of training!) Do what you want to and can do. If something hurts, knock it off. If you get tired, go home. But remember to come back. Fitness builds in increments that follow rest. You're far more likely to experience a breakthrough than a breakdown. And keep records so you can track your progress. It's a big boost to know that you can go farther and do more than you could do a month before.

Put the workouts into your schedule as though they were business appointments for you to keep. If you use a calendar or a day planner, log those workouts in ink. Jealously guard that time you've carved out of your day for your program. Before you know it, the workouts will be habit, and time you'll look forward to. And the people around you will eventually get used to your absences and understand that disappearing a few times a week is yielding enormous benefits in all realms of your life.

Make the decision *once* to work out according to your whole training schedule, so you won't have to renegotiate with yourself every day. Here's what we mean. Decide that you're going to work out every day the schedule puts an activity on your calendar (unless you're sick, injured, or experiencing one of the warning signs of overtraining). Avoid saying, "I'll work out today." When you put the plan on a daily basis, you have to revisit the decision every day. That gives you too many opportunities to make up excuses. When you've already decided to do it on schedule, the agreement is a done deal.

Even the most seasoned athlete will tell you that the hardest part of the workout often is getting out the door. To go or not to go is a bloody battle privately waged in your own head. Here's how to win the battle by tricking that part of your brain shrieking for you to forget about the workout and revert to old bad habits: tackle the problem in stages. Forget about getting to your workout. That's obviously causing you major conflict. Do one simple thing. Put away whatever you're doing. That's all. Now put on your workout clothes. That's all. Get your equipment together and put it next to the door. That's all. Pour yourself a frosty bottle of water. That's all. Open the front door. That's all.

Step out. That's all. Close the door behind you. That's all. Now you're out the door and ready to roll. If you choose to turn back at this point, there's something very wrong. But ninety-nine times out of a hundred, you will have successfully quieted your own objections. After all, what was there to object to? A few small tasks, nonchalantly carried out? No conflict there! Now, go work out.

Find a friend with whom you can share your workout. Not only will you have a wonderful time, but you'll discover that a friend can keep you on schedule. Many people find that although they'll consider canceling their own workouts, they are less willing to break an appointment with someone who's waiting for them. Loyalty and manners almost always win out over personal sloth. In negotiating your workout schedule with a friend, make sure you both agree to be in place on time, every time. Avoid building in a lot of loopholes and acceptable excuses. Nothing is more useless than a plan so sloppy that neither of you feels compelled to honor it.

There are a lot of reasons for sticking to your program. Frankly, the older you are, the less time you have to "get back around to it" when you quit the program. Also, we know that even a short layoff will result in your losing strength and conditioning. After you've worked hard, you don't want to undo all the good you've done. But most of all, you deserve the benefits of glowing good health.

Remember, it's never too late for fitness, but you've waited long enough. Let's get started.

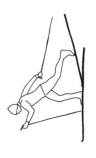

Index

Get in Shape—And Stay in Shape—the Wharton Way!

The Whartons' Stretch Book:
59 Stretches for Over 55 Different Sports and Everyday Activities

Featuring the Breakthrough Method of Active-Isolated Stretching

Whether you're a serious competitor or a weekend warrior, proper stretching before and after your workout can improve your performance, increase your flexibility, help prevent injury, and make you feel better. Active-Isolated Stretching, a ground-breaking technique, developed by researchers, coaches, and trainers and pioneered by Phil and Jim Wharton, is a simple yet revolutionary technique that delivers outstanding results. This bestselling book offers fully illustrated, easy-to-follow stretches for all body zones, with coaches' tips for over 55 sports and activities, from running, tennis, aerobics, and skiing to driving, sitting at a desk, and keyboarding.

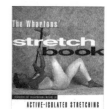

ISBN: 0-8129-2623-4

$15.00

The Whartons' Strength Book:
35 Lifts for Over 55 Different Sports and Everyday Activities

Featuring the Revolutionary Active-Isolated Technique

Active-Isolated Strength Training is a remarkably easy and effective way to tone up, lose weight, rehabilitate from an injury, reshape a sagging waistline, regain lost vitality, or build muscles. This fully illustrated guide will help you create a personal training program backed by sound scientific principles and specifically tailored to your fitness goals and favorite sports. You'll learn 35 simple lifts, the 7 myths of strength training, how to make your own no-cost/low-cost home gym, and workout prescriptions for more than 50 sports and activities, from running, swimming, and cycling to keyboarding and heavy lifting.

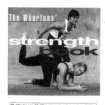

ISBN: 0-8129-2929-2

$15.00

Available from Three Rivers Press wherever books are sold.

THREE RIVERS PRESS
NEW YORK